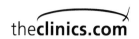

CLINICS IN GERIATRIC MEDICINE

Pain Management

GUEST EDITOR
Howard S. Smith, MD

May 2008 • Volume 24 • Number 2

SAUNDERS

An Imprint of Elsevier, Inc.
PHILADELPHIA   LONDON   TORONTO   MONTREAL   SYDNEY   TOKYO

W.B. SAUNDERS COMPANY
A Division of Elsevier Inc.

Elsevier, Inc. • 1600 John F. Kennedy Blvd., Suite 1800 • Philadelphia, PA 19103-2899

http://www.theclinics.com

CLINICS IN GERIATRIC MEDICINE
May 2008
Editor: Lisa Richman

Volume 24, Number 2
ISSN 0749-0690
ISBN-13: 978-1-4160-6051-2
ISBN-10: 1-4160-6051-0

The ideas and opinions expressed in the *Clinics in Geriatric Medicine* do not necessarily reflect those of the Publisher. The Publisher does not assume any responsibility for any injury and/or damage to persons or property arising out of or related to any use of the material contained in this periodical. The reader is advised to check the appropriate medical literature and the product information currently provided by the manufacturer of each drug to be administered to verify the dosage, the method and duration of administration, or contraindications. It is the responsibility of the treating physician or other health care professional, relying on independent experience and knowledge of the patient, to determine drug dosages and the best treatment for the patient. Mention of any product in this issue should not be construed as endorsement by the contributors, editors, or the Publisher of the product of manufacturers' claims.

Clinics in Geriatric Medicine (ISSN 0749-0690) is published quarterly by Elsevier Inc., 360 Park Avenue South, New York, NY 10010-1710. Months of issue are February, May, August, and November. Business and Editorial Offices: 1600 John F. Kennedy Blvd., Suite 1800, Philadelphia, PA 191023-2899. Customer Service Office: 6277 Sea Harbor Drive, Orlando, FL 32887-4800. Periodicals postage paid at New York, NY, and additional mailing offices. Subscription prices is $189.00 per year (US individuals), $327.00 per year (US institutions), $246.00 per year (Canadian individuals), $398.00 per year (Canadian institutions), $246.00 per year (foreign individuals) and $398.00 per year (foreign institutions). Foreign air speed delivery is included in all *Clinics* subscription prices. All prices are subject to change without notice. POSTMASTER: Send address changes to *Clinics in Geriatric Medicine*, Elsevier Periodicals Customer Service, 6277 Sea Harbor Drive, Orlando, FL 32887-4800. **Customer Service: 1-800-654-2452 (US). From outside of the United States, call 1-407-563-6020. Fax: 1-407-363-9661. E-mail: JournalsCustomerService-usa@elsevier.com.**

Clinics in Geriatric Medicine is covered in *Index Medicus, EMBASE/Excerpta Medica, Current Contents/ Clinical Medicine (CC/CM)*, and the *Cumulative Index to Nursing & Allied Health Literature.*

Printed in the United States of America.

GUEST EDITOR

HOWARD S. SMITH, MD, Academic Director of Pain Management, Department of Anesthesiology, Albany Medical College, Albany, New York

CONTRIBUTORS

KAREN BJORO, PhD(c), RN, Doctoral student, College of Nursing, The University of Iowa, Iowa City, Iowa; and Department of Research, Nursing Unit, Ulleval University Hospital, Oslo, Norway

PATRICIA BRUCKENTHAL, PhD, RN, ANP-BC, Clinical Associate Professor, Department of Adult and Family Health Nursing, School of Nursing, Stony Brook University, Stony Brook; Nurse Practitioner, Pain and Headache Treatment Center, North Shore/Long Island Jewish Health System, Manhasset; and Nurse Practitioner, Department of Neurology, Pain Management Services, North Shore/Long Island Jewish Medical Center, New Hyde Park, New York

ADRIAN CRISTIAN, MD, Associate Professor, Department of Rehabilitation Medcine, Mount Sinai School of Medicine, New York; Department of Rehabilitation Medicine, James J. Peters Veterans Affairs Medical Center, Bronx, New York

GLENN DEANE, PhD, Associate Professor, Department of Sociology, and Director of Public Infrastructure Core, Center for Social and Demographic Analysis, University at Albany, State University of New York, Albany, New York

KRISTINA G. GAUD, BS, Research Associate, Translational Pain Research, Department of Neurosurgery, University of Rochester School of Medicine and Dentistry, Rochester, New York

SAILA K. HARJU, MEd, Department of Psychology, University of Joensuu, Joensuu, Finland

KEELA HERR, PhD, RN, FAAN, AGSF, Professor and Chair, Adult and Gerontology, College of Nursing, The University of Iowa, Iowa City, Iowa

KENNETH L. KIRSH, PhD, Assistant Professor, Pharmacy Practice and Science, University of Kentucky, Lexington, Kentucky

ELIZABETH DEMERS LAVELLE, MD, Cleveland Clinic Foundation; Department of Anesthesiology, Cleveland Clinic, Cleveland, Ohio

WILLIAM F. LAVELLE, MD, Department of Orthopaedic Surgery, The Cleveland Clinic Foundation, Cleveland Clinic Center for Spine Health, Cleveland, Ohio

JOHN D. MARKMAN, MD, Director, Neuromedicine Pain Management Center, and Director, Translational Pain Research, Department of Neurosurgery, University of Rochester School of Medicine and Dentistry, Rochester, New York

GARY McCLEANE, MD, Consultant in Pain Management, Rampark Pain Centre, Lurgan, Northern Ireland, United Kingdom

EWAN McNICOL, BSPharm, MS, Pain Research, Education, and Policy, Pharmacist and Researcher, Tufts–New England Medical Center, Boston, Massachusetts

LISA J. NORELLI, MD, MPH, MRCPsych, Assistant Professor, Department of Psychiatry, Albany Medical College; and Chief of Psychiatry, Capital District Psychiatric Center, Albany, New York

HYON SCHNEIDER, MD, Department of Rehabilitation Medicine, The Mount Sinai Medical Center, New York, New York

HOWARD S. SMITH, MD, Director of Pain Management, Department of Anesthesiology, Albany Medical Center, Albany, New York

SCOTT A. STRASSELS, PharmD, PhD, BCPS, Assistant Professor, Division of Pharmacy Practice, University of Texas at Austin College of Pharmacy, Austin, Texas

ROSY SULEMAN, PharmD, Regional Scientific Associate Director, Novartis Pharmaceuticals Corporation, Carlsbad, California

CONTENTS

challenging for clinicians. The overarching goal of pain assessment in the elderly is to provide successful pain management. This article provides the clinician with the foundation to perform a successful pain assessment for older adults who are able to communicate by self-report. This provides a comprehensive base on which to build a relevant plan of care.

The inability of nonverbal older adults to communicate pain represents a major barrier to pain assessment and treatment. This article focuses on nonverbal older adult populations with dementia, delirium, and severe critical illness. A comprehensive approach to pain assessment is advocated encompassing multiple sources of information. Selected behavioral tools for nonverbal pain assessment are critiqued. Although there are tools with promise, there is currently no standardized behavioral tool that may be recommended for broad adoption in clinical practice and continued concerted effort to this end is needed.

Older patients who have pain present unique challenges for clinicians. On the one hand, care must be taken to treat the pain aggressively while avoiding hampering the patient with excessive side effects, such as drowsiness, nausea and vomiting, and constipation. On the other hand, the clinician must be aware of the growing problem of prescription drug abuse and assess whether or not the patient or his or her family is at risk. Indeed, the concern for assessment is not solely centered on the patient but also extends to the family and extended support network, which may or may not have the patient's best interests at heart when it comes to pain medications. Supposing that addiction and abuse are solely the purview of the young is no longer acceptable, and we have the burden of assessing for problematic behavior while also trying to convince some patients that they would benefit from pain medicine.

Pain is a universal part of being human, and yet, there is ample evidence that many people from all backgrounds, stages of life, and levels of health care experience receive less than optimal treatment of their pain. This article reviews the pharmacotherapy of pain in older adults, with a focus on salicylates, nonsteroidal anti-inflammatory drugs, and opioids.

Topical Analgesic Agents

Gary McCleane

Pain processing and transmission are achieved by a complex interaction of pathways and processes. Those parts of the process with peripheral representation may be amenable to therapeutic intervention by systemic administration to achieve a peripheral effect or by local application, including local topical administration to the skin overlying the painful area. Advantages include high level of patient acceptance, ease of administration, avoidance of systemic side effects, and reduced drug-drug interactions. Those drugs with topical analgesic effects include those with specific topical analgesic indication and others in which no such indication exists but that may offer a chance of pain therapy at reduced risk.

Role of Rehabilitation Medicine in the Management of Pain in Older Adults

Hyon Schneider and Adrian Cristian

Pain management may play an important role in contributing to optimal quality of life in the elderly population. Pain lowers overall quality of life in part by decreasing function and by amplifying the psychologicic stress of aging. A comprehensive, multidisciplinary approach to pain management, with preservation and restoration of function in older adults, is the cornerstone of an effective pain management program.

Behavioral Approaches to Pain Management in the Elderly

Lisa J. Norelli and Saila K. Harju

Pain is a complex phenomenon, influenced by many individual and external factors, and may be experienced differently with age. The detrimental health and social effects of chronic pain are well known. Age-related disorders, such as dementia, may interfere with the communication of pain. Health care provider bias and cultural expectations also may be barriers to the recognition and management of pain in the elderly. A multidisciplinary and multimodal approach in older adults is essential to effective assessment and management. Behavioral approaches to pain should be considered and incorporated into treatment where appropriate.

CLINICS IN
GERIATRIC
MEDICINE

Clin Geriatr Med 24 (2008) xi–xii

ELSEVIER
SAUNDERS

Preface

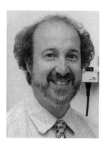

Howard S. Smith, MD
Guest Editor

Pain and suffering remain among the most terrible symptoms that some older adults may experience as they grow older. It is not infrequent to hear older adults giving this advice to younger adults: do not grow old. One significant reason that some older adults may feel this way is the experience of constant, severe pain that may occur in the geriatric population. In this issue of *Clinics in Geriatric Medicine*, readers are exposed to a broad spectrum of available evaluation and management strategies.

Severe, constant pain and suffering can contribute to social, emotional, and physical isolation for older adults, with resultant significant decreases in quality of life. Elderly patients may complain of similar physical symptoms with similar intensities yet report markedly different perceptions of quality of life. Different levels of distress from similar degrees of pain may stem from variations in many factors, including culture and environment, coping mechanisms, experiences, support systems, beliefs, perceptions of the meaning of pain, and spirituality. A particular concern that may make the treatment of pain in older adults even more challenging is that the geriatric population is generally more susceptible to adverse effects of therapy than their younger counterparts. Clinicians must make special efforts to carefully weigh the risk-to-benefit ratio of each treatment decision with older patients before proceeding with therapy. In older adults, it may be especially challenging to provide optimal analgesia with minimal significant adverse effects. When addressing pain in older persons, it seems to be particularly useful (as long as the patient is agreeable) to involve a patient's

0749-0690/08/$ - see front matter © 2008 Elsevier Inc. All rights reserved.
doi:10.1016/j.cger.2007.12.012   *geriatric.theclinics.com*

significant other or caregivers and family in some of the assessment and management processes and techniques.

When treating older persons for persistent pain, it also seems particularly important that health care providers attempt to use evidence-based approaches that provide optimal outcomes not only for pain relief but also for other domains (eg, optimal quality of life and optimal physical, emotional, social, and cognitive functioning). In this issue, the first two articles provide an overview of pain in older adults and discuss differences in age-related pain perception. The next three articles focus on state-of-the-art assessment strategies and other issues in the evaluation of older persons with pain. The following six articles concentrate on analgesic treatment strategies for persistent pain in older adults.

Clinicians remain limited in their ability to pinpoint the molecular mechanisms of pain in older adults; however, it is hoped that this issue will help health care providers to better assess and evaluate pain complaints and their impact on older persons in efforts to optimally manage persistent pain.

Howard S. Smith, MD
Department of Anesthesiology
Albany Medical College
47 New Scotland Avenue, MC-131
Albany, New York 12208, USA

E-mail address: SmithH@mail.amc.edu

ELSEVIER
SAUNDERS

Clin Geriatr Med 24 (2008) 185–201

CLINICS IN
GERIATRIC
MEDICINE

Overview of Pain Management in Older Persons

Glenn Deane, PhD[a],*, Howard S. Smith, MD[b]

[a]Department of Sociology, University at Albany, State University of New York,
Albany, NY 12222, USA
[b]Department of Anesthesiology, MC-131, Albany Medical Center,
47 New Scotland Avenue, Albany, NY 12208, USA

The purpose of this introductory article is to situate the social and demographic context of pain management in older adults. It starts by summarizing the composition and trajectory of older adult population in the United States. The authors then comment on the research literature on pain prevalence and management. While acknowledging that excellent reviews of pain in older persons research are brought together in Gibson and Weiner [1], it appears that epidemiologic pain research remains in its infancy. Aside from a universal recognition that pain is associated with psychologic and physical disability, a source of individual suffering, familial distress, and consumption of community resources, there is strikingly little agreement in even the most basic descriptions of pain prevalence. This article summarizes representative literature on the age and sex composition of pain among older adults and considers sources of assessment bias that likely lead to the conflicting descriptions of prevalence. Likewise there is a comprehensive literature on pain management in older adults. The authors briefly review this literature, citing evidence on how pain affects quality of life beyond the local site of injury and commenting on how the difficulties of assessment and suboptimal treatment undermine universal pain management guidelines. They conclude by enumerating the wide range of treatments that are available, and acceptable, to older adults.

Who is at risk now and in the future?: aging in the United States

Based on short-form data from Census 2000, the 65-and-older population comprised 35 million people, representing 12.4% of the 281.4 million people

---

* Corresponding author.
 E-mail address: gdd@albany.edu (G. Deane).

enumerated on April 1, 2000. Within this group, 18.5 million people, representing 53% of the elderly were in the age group 65 to 74; 12.3 million (35%)
were aged 75 to 84, and 4.2 million (12%) were aged 85 and over.[1] In 1990,
there were 31.1 million elderly Americans, but proportionately, the 65 and
older population decreased slightly between 1990 and 2000, as the 31.1
million elderly represented 12.5% of the total 1990 United States population. Persons aged 85 and older numbered 3 million in 1990, about 9.6%
of the elderly population and about 1.2% of the total 1990 United States
population. America's most populous states are also those with the largest
elderly populations, with California, Florida, New York, Pennsylvania,
and Texas leading the way. Regionally, the greatest increase in the elderly
population was in western and southeastern coastal States. Although
California has the largest number of elderly, Florida has the nation's largest
proportion of elderly. Several Midwestern states, including Iowa, South
Dakota, North Dakota, Nebraska, and Kansas, have a higher proportion
of elderly than for the total United States.

The longer run trend in aging is more revealing. In 1900, there were
3.1 million elderly in the United States, representing about 1 in 25 Americans. There were about 122,000 persons aged 85 and older, only a fraction
of 1% of the total population. By 2020, the elderly population is projected
to reach 54 million persons, representing a growth rate from 1990 more than
double that of the total population. About one in six Americans would be
elderly. Persons aged 85 and older are expected to number 6.5 million in
2020, more than double the number in 1990. The number of Americans
100 years old and over could increase eightfold from 1990. Interim state
population projections show 26 states are expected to more than double
their elderly populations between 2000 and 2030 [4]. Alaska, Arizona, and
Nevada are projected to more than triple their population of those aged
65 years and over.

Beginning in 2011, the first members of the Baby Boom (the cohort born
in 1946) will reach age 65. In 2050, the final phase of the gerontological
explosion will be reached. Census projections place the number of elderly
at about 79 million, more than double the current number. About one in
five Americans would be aged 65 and older. The population aged 65 to 74
years old is expected to reach its peak of 38 million in 2030, then decline
to 35 million in 2050. This is still almost double the number in Census
2000. The population 75 to 84 years old is expected to peak at 29 million
in 2040, then decrease to 26 million in 2050. The oldest-old population
(referring to the 85-and-over age group) is expected to increase more than
fourfold from the 4.2 million enumerated in Census 2000 to the projected
population of 17.7 million in 2050, with this age group more than doubling

---

[1] The population statistics presented in this section are extracted from two U.S. Census
Bureau reports, "We the people: aging in the United States," issued in December 2004 [2],
and "We, the American elderly," issued in September 1993 [3].

from the expected 8.4 million in 2030 to 2050. In 2050, the oldest-old would account for about 5% of the total United States population. The significance of the oldest-old population is also revealed by the Census Bureau's projected long-term trend in the ratio of persons 85 and older per persons ages 50 to 64 years old. These projections were developed to give a sense of elderly survivorship for older adults. The Census Bureau refers to this as the "parent support ratio." In 1950, there were three persons 85 years old and over for every 100 persons aged 50 to 64. By 2000, this ratio was 10:100, by 2030 the parent support ratio is expected to reach 15 and by 2050 the ratio will be 27. In other words, about one person aged 85 and older for every three persons between the ages of 50 to 64.

In 2000, the sex ratio (the number of males per 100 women) for the total United States population was 96. In the 65-and-over population, the sex ratio was only 70, with 20.6 million women compared with 14.4 million men. The age group-specific sex ratios decline precipitously from 82.4 in the 65 to 74 age group to 64.4 among those aged 75 to 84, and 40.7, less than one male for every two females, at ages 85 and older. Although the difference between the number of men and women grows with advancing age, because of the longer life expectancy of women, in the future, mortality differences between men and women may narrow. As evidence, in 1990, elderly women outnumbered elderly men three to two, with 18.6 million women aged 65 and older compared with 12.5 million men. Still, the health, social, and economic problems of the elderly will be gendered disproportionately.

In 2000, 56% of the 65 and over population were married, 32% widowed, and 7% divorced. Not surprisingly, the percentage married decreased with age (66% of those 65 to 74 years old were married compared with less than 31% of those 85 and older), while the percentage widowed increased steeply among the elderly age groups (20.7% of those 65 to 74 years old to 40.3% of those 75 to 84, to 61.1% of those 85 and older). Most elderly men, however, are married, while most elderly women are not. Elderly men are nearly twice as likely as elderly women to be married; elderly women are more than three times as likely to be widowed. Marital status differs considerably by both age and sex. In the 65 to 74 age group, four-fifths of men compared with half of women are married. At 85 and over, about half of men are married, while four-fifths of women are widowed. In 2000, 28% of the elderly lived alone. Approximately 7.5 million women aged 65 and older lived alone, compared with 2.4 million elderly men. This type of living arrangement increases with age, with 22.1% of those aged 65 to 74 years old living alone compared with 33.7% aged 75 to 84, and 38.9% of those aged 85 and older. It is perhaps more telling to look at living arrangements from the perspective of the Census category "living with others in a household," with 76.1% of the 65 to 74 age group reporting this living arrangement, compared with 60.3% aged 75 to 84 years old, and 39.2% aged 85 and older. The oldest-old are as likely to live alone as to live with others in a household.

About 6% of the elderly live in group quarters, although less than 2% of persons aged 65 to 74 years old have this type of living arrangements. The percentage living in group quarters increases to 6% for the 75 to 84 age group and then to 21.9% for those aged 85 and older. In 1990, 1.6 million elderly persons lived in nursing homes. Nine states (California, Florida, Illinois, Massachusetts, Michigan, New York, Ohio, Pennsylvania, and Texas) had more than 50,000 elderly nursing home residents. About 1.3 million of the 1.6 million (over 81%) nursing home residents were female. Only one in seven elderly living in nursing homes was married; three in five were widowed.

Ten percent of the elderly population in Census 2000 were foreign born, compared with 11% of the total population. In 2000, 13% of the elderly population spoke a language other than English at home, compared with 18% for the total population (aged 5 and older), though about half of the older population who reported speaking a language other than English at home also reported that they spoke English very well. In 1990, about 90% of the elderly reported their race category as white. Census Bureau projections show that, although the number of elderly whites will more than double between 1990 and 2050, the racial and ethnic composition of older Americans will diversify. According to these projections, the number of elderly blacks will nearly quadruple (from 2.5 million in 1990 to 9.4 million in 2050); the number of elderly Hispanics will increase 11-fold from 1990 to 12 million in 2050.

Although the socioeconomic conditions of the elderly decline with age, older Americans do compare favorably with the total population on some characteristics. For example, in 2000 12.4% of the total population lived in poverty. The poverty rate for those aged 65 and over was 9.9%. The percentage of the elderly in poverty increased by age group, with 8.5% of persons 65 to 74 years old in poverty compared with 10.6% of the 75 to 84 age group, and 14.7% of the population 85 years and older. Social security income made an important contribution, as 90% of households with a householder 65 and over received social security income. About one in three households with a householder 65 and over had earnings as a source of income (compared with four out of five of all households), and about half of households with elderly householder reported retirement income. Homeownership rates also decline with age, but the 65 to 74 and 75 to 84 age groups reported much higher homeownership in 2000 than the percentage (66.2%) for all occupied units. Over 77% of elderly householders owned their homes, with homeownership rates of 80.9% for the 65 to 74 age group, 76.6% for persons 75 to 84 years old, and 65.3% for the oldest old.

Median earnings vary by age and sex, as do labor force participation rates. In 2000, the median annual earnings for employed, full-time, year-round workers aged 65 and older was $31,556 for men and $22,511 for women. These earnings can be compared with $37,057 for all male workers and $27,194 for all female workers. Although median earnings for men and women ages 65 to 74 are the highest among elderly workers, earnings reported in the Census 2000 did not differ appreciably among the 75 to 84 and 85 and older age groups. As expected, the labor force participation rates of elderly men and women (18.4% and 9.7%, respectively, for ages 65 and older) are much below the total population (70.7% and 57.5% for all men and women, respectively). Labor force participation rates decline precipitously for older males and females. The educational attainment of elderly Americans is also well below that of the total population, but the biggest differential resides in the percentage not completing high school rather than among the higher attainment categories "high school graduate," "some college or associate's degree," or "bachelor's degree of more." According to Census 2000, 19.6% of the total population ages 25 and older reported that they had not completed high school, compared with 34.5% of persons aged 65 and over. Nearly half of people 85 and over had not completed high school. The percentage reporting that their highest educational attainment was a high school degree was 28.6% for the total population, 32% for all elderly, 32.8% for persons ages 65 to 74 years old, 32.5% for the 75 to 84 age group, and 26.7% for persons 85 years and older.

Diversity and growth describe America's elderly [2]. The elderly is a commonly used term for persons aged 65 and older, but the elderly are a heterogeneous population. Growth is another significant factor when addressing the elderly population. Population projections show that different age groups will peak in size, and account for different proportions of the total elderly population, at different times in the not too distant future. If assessment and pain management must be tailored in different ways to different groups, the characterizations of the elderly given here suggest caution. Because the elderly are increasing in number and living longer, America has begun to experience cultural change that comes with an aging society; it would be naive to believe that the future of pain management will be unaffected by that change.

Disability in older ages

In 2000, 42% of the population 65 and over reported some type of long-lasting condition or disability. The Census 2000 asked about various sensory, physical, and mental disabilities, and disabilities causing difficulty giving self-care and difficulty going outside the home.[2] Disability in each category is much higher among the elderly than in the total population, and disability increases with age. For example, 8.2% of the total population reported a physical disability (defined as "long lasting, substantial limitation on one

---

[2] For more information on disability from the Census 2000, see the Census report "Disability: 2000" issued March 2003 [5].

or more basic physical activities, such as walking, climbing stairs, reaching, lifting, or carrying"), compared with 21.5% of the 65– to 74-year-old population, 32.7% of those 75 to 84 years old, and 53.1% of persons ages 85 and older. Over one in three persons in the 85 and older age group reported a sensory disability (eg, blindness or deafness); almost 30% of the oldest old reported a mental disability. Twenty-seven percent reported difficulty giving self-care (eg, dressing, bathing, getting around the inside of the home), and almost half reported disabilities causing difficulty going outside the home. In all categories except physical disability, the percentage reporting disability more than doubled from those 75 to 84 years old to the 85 and older group.

Unintentional falls are an important source of disability and a common occurrence among older adults. According to a Centers for Disease Control and Prevention's (CDC) Morbidity and Mortality Weekly Report [6], unintentional falls affect approximately 30% of persons aged 65 and older each year. In 2003, 13,700 elderly persons died from falls, and 1.8 million were treated in emergency departments for nonfatal injuries from falls. Falls cause most hip fractures, which often result in long-term disability and may require admission to a nursing home for a year or more. Between 2001 and 2005, the overall rate of nonfatal injuries from falls did not change, although the rate of hospitalizations for hip fractures decreased. The rate of nonfatal falls for women aged 65 and older was approximately 1.5 times the rate for men. The CDC did not find meaningful differences in the rates for non-Hispanic whites and blacks.

The causal relationship between pain and falls runs in both directions. Self-reported functional ability and pain have a modest independent association with physiologic predictors of the risk of falls [7]. An especially important location of pain in older adults is the foot/ankle region. Foot and ankle problems may be associated with impaired balance and impaired functional ability, which in turn may lead to increased risk of fall in older adults [8]. Menz and colleagues have confirmed the high prevalence of disabling foot pain in the elderly [8–10]. In 2001, Menz and colleagues [9,10] performed foot problem assessments on 135 community-dwelling older persons in conjunction with clinical tests of balance and functional ability. Eighty-seven percent of the sample had at least one foot problem including: hallus valgus, which may lead to gait instability and falls [10], plantar hyperkeratosis, lesser digital deformity, and lesser digital lesions [9]. Older people at risk of falling should be advised to wear shoes indoors where possible [11]. Menz and colleagues [12] studied a sample of 301 community-dwelling people (117 men, 184 women) aged between 70 and 95 years (mean 77.2, standard deviation 4.9), who also underwent a clinical assessment of foot problems. Their findings confirmed the high prevalence of disabling foot pain in older people, and suggest that the Manchester Foot Pain and Disability Index (MFPDI) is a suitable tool for assessing foot pain in this population [12].

Prevalence of pain in older adults

Research on the prevalence of pain in adult populations is in agreement that pain is a common and important deterrent to quality of life in older people. It is important to recognize, however, that that is apparently where agreement ends. The context of this article is one in which prior research shows little consensus concerning the level, population composition, and age trajectory of pain.

In establishing the background and significance for guidelines for managing persistent pain in older persons, the American Geriatrics Society (AGS) Panel on Persistent Pain in Older Persons (2002) places pain prevalence at one in five older Americans. Citing a recent Harris survey [13], the AGS panel reports 18% of people 65 years and over are taking analgesic medications regularly (several times a week or more), and 63% of those had taken prescription pain medications for more than 6 months [14]. A review of 11 studies that contain sufficient detail to allow comparison of overall pain rates across a wide age range by Gibson and Helme [15,16] places prevalence at 13% to 88% among the ages of 65 to 74, 29% to 86% among those aged 75 to 84, and 40% to 79% among the 85 and older population. Brattberg and colleagues [17], Crook and colleagues [18], Magni and colleagues [19], and von Korff and colleagues [20] all report pain prevalence at the lower end of these distributions. Conversely, Miro and colleagues [21] report 3-month prevalence of any pain at 73.5% among respondents aged 65 and older. Brochet and colleagues [22] find prevalence of 71.5% in the 65 and older population. Roy and Thomas [23] put prevalence at 80% among people 65 to 74 years old, and Brattberg and colleagues [24] report prevalence at approximately 75% of those older than 75.

Much of the discrepancy in prevalence can be traced to differences in length of reporting period and, to a lesser extent, to degrees of pain severity and local definitions of pain (eg, head, joint, abdomen). One therefore would expect lower prevalence in Crook and colleagues, because they ask about "often troubled by pain" during the last 2 weeks, while Brattberg and colleagues [24] use 12 month prevalence of "mild-to-severe" pain. von Korff and colleagues report separate prevalence for head, chest, and abdominal pain in last 6 months, while Roy and Thomas ask about all types of pain. Still, it is hard to reconcile why Sternbach [25] finds 12-month head pain prevalence of 50% among those 65 to 85 years old, while von Korff and colleagues report that only 1% of this same age group cite head pain during a 6-month prevalence period.

There also is little agreement concerning the age trajectory of prevalence, duration, severity, and compositional differences in pain prevalence. It has been argued that the prevalence of pain increases with age but declines somewhat after age 60 [26,27], but other research shows either no difference among older adults [21,28,29], slight increase [19,22] or substantial increase [18,30]. Brattberg and colleagues [17] report an increase in prevalence at older ages for men, but a decrease for women. Brochet and colleagues found an increase in prevalence only for women. Jakobsson and colleagues show much higher prevalence for women in the oldest age group (90 and older); Miro and colleagues find higher prevalence for women regardless of age. Helme and Gibson [27,31] report no evidence of an increase in duration or severity at older ages. Although Miro and colleagues find no age difference in intensity, they describe a positive relationship between age and duration of pain (with women reporting an earlier onset of pain). Jakobsson and colleagues show severity of pain is worse among the oldest old (85 And older).

Overview of impact of pain in older adults

Research has shown that the effect of pain may be multimodal, affecting quality of life far beyond the local region of injury. Some have proposed that the number of sites of pain may be more important than the precise location [32]. Although this insight is undoubtedly of great significance, there is another reason to think beyond regional pain conditions. The comorbidity of pain and psychologic distress is well-documented. The feeling of loneliness is the single most important predictor of psychologic state of distress in older persons [33]. Findings also suggest that psychosocial factors/barriers have the strongest influence in the etiology of loneliness [34]. In a cohort of 800 older adults followed annually for up to 4 years, lonely persons were more than twice as likely to develop an Alzheimer's disease-like dementia syndrome than were those who were not lonely, even after controlling for level of social isolation [35]. Cacioppo and colleagues [36] found that loneliness appears to be a specific risk factor for depressive symptoms and that loneliness and depressive symptoms can act in a synergistic fashion to diminish well-being in middle-aged and older adults. Factors that have been found to increase levels of loneliness among older persons residing in a nursing home include lack of intimate relationships, increased dependency, and loss [37].

Furthermore, experiences of existential loneliness or isolation may be triggered or promoted by the health care team. Patients who are in need of support (especially in the palliative care setting) when—left alone, avoided, treated disrespectfully or talked to/touched in a nonempathetic manner—may voice feelings of: "being alone in a world of one's own," "feeling invisible," or "feelings of being treated like an animal" [38]. Drageset [39], using a survey design on 113 subjects aged 65 to101 years living in nursing homes, concluded that activities of daily living (eg, feeding, going to the toilet, transferring from bed to chair, dressing, and bathing) and contact with a social network have a statistical effect on a low level of social loneliness.

Although there is a dearth of large well-designed studies on pain and loneliness, there appears to be a significant interaction between loneliness and pain [40–42]. Eisenberger and colleagues [43] found that lower pain unpleasantness thresholds were associated with greater self-reported social distress in response to social rejection conditions, providing support for the hypothesis that pain distress and social distress share neurocognitive substrates.

Cole and colleagues [44] tracked a group of 153 people in their 50s and 60s using responses to the University of California, Los Angeles (UCLA) Loneliness Scale. Cole and colleagues studied DNA from the white blood cells of eight people who scored in the top 15th percentile of loneliness and six who scored in the bottom 15th percentile. Of the 22,000 human genes, 209 were expressed abnormally in the very lonely group. Promoter-based bioinformatic analyses revealed underexpression of genes bearing anti-inflammatory glucocorticoid response elements [GREs] ($P = .032$), and overexpression of genes bearing response elements for proinflammatory NF-kB/Rel, providing a functional genomic explanation for elevated risk of inflammatory disease in individuals who experience chronically high levels of subjection social isolation.

Research also has demonstrated the comorbidity of pain and sleeplessness. The relevance of sleep disturbances increases with age [45,46]. Twenty percent to 45% of older persons report dissatisfaction with sleep, and the elderly in institutionalized settings have reported even higher rates [47]. Aging is associated with a decrease in slow-wave sleep, spindle counts, and arousal thresholds, with an increase in transient arousal thresholds [48]. Pain is among the best predictors of sleep disturbances among older adults [49].

Older persons who have pain are almost twice as likely to have sleep disturbances as older persons without pain [30]. Achieving analgesia is associated with improved sleep. Thus, it appears that improved pain leads to improved sleep, and improved sleep leads to improved pain. Therefore, older people who have pain should be evaluated for sleep disturbances, and if sleep disturbances are identified, they should be treated. In older persons, nonpharmacologic interventions (eg, cognitive–behavioral therapy [CBT]) to improve sleep may be the best first-line therapeutic options to address sleep disturbances.

Another means in which chronic pain can detract significantly from quality of life is by means of disruption of attention [50]. Dick and Rashiq found that it is likely a specific cognitive mechanism, the maintenance of the memory trace that is affected by chronic pain during task performance.

The problem of pain assessment

It is clear that the basic facts about pain prevalence still need to be settled. Prior research is tainted by the lack of statistical power because of small sample size, inconsistencies in fundamental definitions and measurement, and sample selection biases. The effects of survey design and content on the understanding of the health and functioning of older person now are understood [51,52]. Corder and Manton provide an excellent review of the analytic issues in studying morbidity of the elderly. All of their points are directly applicable to the pain prevalence literature cited previously.

Corder and Manton argue that despite the increasing need for information, most currently available data resources are limited, because existing national health surveys were not designed explicitly for older populations. They have both sample design and measurement limitations that become more severe for the oldest old population, because the ability to collect high-quality data and to maintain high response rates is correlated with age-related change in functional impairment and the intensity of health service needs. The authors argue that a failure to relate changes in the distribution of health characteristics to individual-level changes has produced serious biases in studies of the elderly. First, if the prevalence of morbidity is related to age in a population, random samples of populations at each age will reflect those differences in prevalence with age. The age trajectory of that prevalence is not the same as the rate of physiologic aging in an individual. Second, mortality selection operating between the survey dates or, for rapidly occurring events for the oldest old, within the period of field work, may introduce a bias in parameter estimates representing individual changes. That bias increases with the amount of mortality and the degree of individual heterogeneity. Thus the measurement of health and functioning for individuals must be adequate to estimate transition parameters adjusted for both mortality selection and the emergent effects of latent diseases and their effects on individual functioning.

The authors conclude that panel studies using list samples, with health service data drawn from administrative records and heavy oversampling of the oldest old, appeared to be the most cost-effective design. The authors also conclude that specialized surveys of the elderly, using current household field procedures and interviewing methods produce accurate and reliable data, can achieve the same levels of statistical confidence for estimators at lower cost and are preferable to further increasing the administrative and analytic complexity of large multipurpose studies. The designs that worked best had instrumentation on health and functioning that was substantively rich and thus permitted the use of multivariate procedures to improve reliability and to define multiple dimensions of health and functional status [51].

Accurate assessment of the level, duration, severity, composition, and age trajectory of pain is a necessary precursor to pain management. It is difficult, and perhaps dangerous, to set guidelines for pain management in the absence of basic knowledge. In their introduction to the "Epidemiology of Pain in Older Persons," Jones and Macfarlane [32] note several problems that make it difficult to define and measure pain for epidemiologic research. If pain is defined as a subjective phenomenon, analysts must rely on self-report or clinical diagnosis. The reporting of pain, however, is filtered through individual and cultural influences, and only a small proportion of sufferers seek medical intervention. As evidence, Jones and Macfarlane cite a large prospective cohort study in the United Kingdom that found that although a third of the study subjects reported a new episode of lower back pain (LBP), only 4% consulted their family practitioner about their symptoms. Even when medical intervention is sought, clinical diagnosis of even basic fitness is not unambiguous. In older persons, for example, the 6-minute walk distance (6MWD) is a basic diagnostic test, but its measure is conditional on multiple physiologic, psychologic, and health factors [53]. The 6MWD seems to provide an indicator of overall mobility and physical function in the geriatric population rather than a specific measure of cardiovascular fitness [53].

Jones and Macfarlane also target the fluidity of the definition of prevalence as a significant problem in pain epidemiology. It is understood that prevalence refers to the proportion of persons who have disease within the population of interest at a given point or period in time. Small differences in definitions of duration (eg, 1 month prevalence, 6 month prevalence, 1 year prevalence) or the etiology of occurrence (mild, persistent, severe) or location (neck, LBP, any), however, can result in large changes in the estimates of pain occurrence.

Overview of pain management in older adults

If one sets aside the possibility that prevalence could be too low to constitute a management issue, uncovering the direction and magnitude of change is a necessary prerequisite to management. For example, if prevalence truly decreases at older ages, then it is productive to determine whether that change is a function of change in nociceptive pathways or whether the elderly deemphasize or misattribute pain because of the aging process and accruement of significant life events such as death of a spouse, loss of independence, and mobility. Helme and Gibson [16] write that it is equally important to determine the extent to which selection bias may be at source. For instance, older persons who have painful disease may be sequestered into institutional care, thereby reducing pain prevalence estimates among older persons in general population-based samples. The nonresponse rates among the very old in community surveys may be exceptionally high, especially for those who are disabled by disease and hence more likely to suffer from pain. The very oldest also represent a select sample of survivors, and these individuals may experience less pain-causing disease.

Here are reviewed two sources of information on pain management in older adults, (1) the AGS clinical practice guideline [14] and its critiques [54,55] and (2) empiric and theoretic research [56–58].

Certainly one of the primary sources on pain management is the guideline composed by the AGS Panel on Persistent Pain in Older Persons. On May 9, 2002, the AGS released a revised update of its 1998 guideline for managing chronic pain in the elderly. The 1998 guideline recommended earlier use of narcotics than is typical for treatment of younger patients because of the significant toxicities associated with nonsteroidal anti-inflammatory drugs (NSAIDs). In addition to raising awareness of the problem of undertreatment of pain, the guideline supported a general movement away from the extreme reluctance of physicians to prescribe narcotics, citing that fear of addiction and other adverse effects does not justify failure to treat severe pain [54].

The revised guideline's goals were developed to provide advice on the assessment and management of persistent pain in frail, vulnerable elders with limited social and financial resources. The panel members who developed the guideline reviewed over 4122 citations and 2089 abstracts in the scientific literature. Despite the large meta-analysis, the panelists acknowledged a serious limitation in the published data, with few randomized trials among older patients and very few longitudinal studies. Thus, many of the recommendations made for treatment of frail, elderly individuals who had persistent pain were not supported by strong, published scientific evidence [54].

The difficulties in providing universal recommendations are immediately evident in the guideline's "assessment of persistent pain." The general principles begin by stating that "the most accurate and reliable evidence of the existence of pain and its intensity is the patient's report. Even patients with mild to moderate cognitive impairment can be assessed with simple questions and screening tools [14]." This statement is undermined only a paragraph later when the document admits "older patients themselves may make accurate pain assessment difficult. They may be reluctant to report pain despite substantial physical or psychologic impairment. Many older people expect pain with aging and do not believe that their pain can be alleviated. Some patients accept pain and suffering as atonement for past actions [14]." The general principles on assessment conclude by advising that "assessment and treatment strategies need to be sensitive to culture and ethnicity, as well as the values and beliefs of individual patients and families. Information from family and other caregivers should also be included in the assessment [14]."

Finucane also notes variability in reporting of pain symptoms, even for cognitively intact patients. Eich and colleagues [59] find that patients who have persistent headaches, reports of past pain were more intense if the individuals were interviewed during a period of serious headache compared with when they were interviewed during a time of milder or no headache. Past pain also was reported to be more severe by patients evidencing increased emotional distress, conflict, and discord in the household [60].

In addition to the complexities of assessment, the provision of quality care and treatment of pain in older adults is equally, if not more, problematic. Burgess and colleagues [58] speculate on how racial and ethnic stereotypes may lead to unintentional provider bias in decisions about pain treatment. In turn, these biases may lead providers to contribute to disparities in pain treatment. In a study of 372 seniors (ages ranged from 66 to 98) enrolled in two managed care organizations, Chodosh and colleagues [56] found that less than 40% of vulnerable patients reported having been screened for pain over a 2-year period. Although this study could not document under-recognition of pain, the authors conclude that the low prevalence of screening (an adequate diagnostic history was documented for only 39% of those presenting with pain) suggests that opportunities to identify chronic pain potentially responsive to treatment often are missed.

The treatment of pain in older adults in general should be multimodal and may be particularly challenging in efforts to abolish pain with minimal adverse effects. Pharmacologic approaches may include: opioids, anti-inflammatory agents (aspirin, nonsteroidal NSAIDs, cyclooxygenase [COX]-2 inhibitors, steroids), acetaminophen, tramadol, muscle relaxants, antidepressants) tricyclic antidepressants (TVAs), selective serotonin norepinephrine reuptake inhibitors (SNRIs), and antiepileptic drugs (AEDs).

Nonpharmacologic approaches are primarily physical medicine approaches, behavioral medicine approaches, and complementary and alternative medicine (CAM) approaches. Physical medicine approaches may include range of motion (ROM) and strengthening exercises, aerobic postural and other exercises, modalities (ice, moist heat), galvanic ultrasound (GUS), transcutaneous electrical nerve stimulation (TENS), myofascial release techniques, manipulative therapy, traction, and functional restorative therapy. Behavioral medicine approaches may include biofeedback (BFB), CBT, hypnosis, relaxation techniques, psychoanalytic therapy, distraction techniques, guided imagery, and progressive muscle relaxation.

Austrian and colleagues [57] surveyed patients aged 70 and older at a community-based geriatric primary care practice who sought treatment for pain from a noncancer cause and found very high percentage indicating interest and willingness to try an exercise program and relaxation methods as pain management strategies. Although only 16% of patients reported current use of exercise, and only 4% were using relaxation methods, over 70% indicated a willingness to try these means of pain management. The study also found that commonly cited barriers to the use of exercise and relaxation methods included time conflicts, transportation, treatment efficacy, and fear of pain or injury.

Increasing numbers of patients, including older patients, appear to be using CAM to alleviate various symptoms and/or symptom distress (eg, pain, nausea, insomnia, dyspnea) [61–66]. Even during the last months of life, significant numbers of nonhospitalized patients used CAM techniques in efforts to achieve symptom palliation [67]. Additionally, it appears that CAM therapies are used widely by patients receiving opioids for chronic pain [68]. CAM approaches may include acupuncture, yoga, tai chi, gi gong herbal therapy meditation, music therapy, massage, reiki/therapeutic touch, and prayer.

Finally, there is also a role for interventional and invasive/surgical procedures in older persons who have persistent pain; however, these options should be considered carefully and fully discussed with the patient/caregiver/family.

Summary

The most recent United States censuses and population projections show that America's elderly are growing in number and diversity. This takes on added importance, because most models of prevalence of pain embrace the notion of age-related change. Citing Andersson and colleagues [26], Jones and Macfarlane [32] discuss four such models. The first holds that pain increases with age and then decreases at older ages (ie, ages 70 and beyond). They suppose that this pain typically has a mechanical etiologic component and possibly is associated with the occupational environment. The second model has pain increasing with age. This model has a mechanical etiologic component but also an association with increasing prevalence of degenerative disease, particularly at older ages. The third model is age-independent pain that (obviously) lacks a mechanical etiologic component (ie, risk factors are constant throughout the life course). Jones and Macfarlane also find some evidence to propose a fourth model that posits a decrease in pain prevalence at older ages. It is not clear whether the trajectory is caused by age-related changes in pain and pain perception, or by changes in pain reporting.

In all but the third model, changes in the size and composition of the elderly will have important consequences for assessment and pain management. As the size and composition of the elderly population changes, strategies for pain management must remain flexible and sensitive to changes in older adults' treatment preferences.

References

[1] Gibson SJ, Weiner DK, editors. Pain in older persons. Seattle (WA): IASP Press; 2005.

[2] Gist YJ, Hetzel LI. We the people: aging in the United States. Census 2000 special reports, US Census Bureau. Issued December 2004. Available at: http://www.census.gov/prod/2004pubs/censr-19.pdf.

[3] Goldstein A, Damon H. We, the American elderly. US Census Bureau. Issued September 1993. Available at: http://www.census.gov/apsd/wepeople/we-9.pdf.

[4] U.S. Census Bureau. Population division, interim state population projections. Tables 3 and 4: interim projections. Internet Release Date: April 21, 2005. Available at: http://www.census.gov/population/www/projections/projectionsagesex.html.

[5] Waldrop J, Stern SM. Disability status: 2000. Census 2000 brief, C2KBR-17. Issued March 2003. Available at: http://www.census.gov/prod/2003pubs/c2kbr-17.pdf.

[6] Stevens JA, Ryan G, Kresnow M. Fatalities and injuries from falls among older adults—United States, 1993–2003 and 2001–2005. MMWR Morb Mortal Wkly Rep 2006;55(45): 1221–4.

[7] Foley SJ, Lord SR, Srikanth V, et al. Falls risk is associated with pain and dysfunction but not radiographic osteoarthritis in older adults: Tasmanian Older Adult Cohort study. Osteoarthritis Cartilage 2006;14:533–9.

[8] Menz HB, Morris ME, Lord SR. Foot and ankle risk factors for falls in older people: a prospective study. J Gerontol A Biol Sci Med Sci 2006;61:866–70.

[9] Menz HB, Lord SR. Foot pain impairs balance and functional ability in community-dwelling older people. J Am Podiatr Med Assoc 2001;91:222–9.

[10] Menz HB, Lord SR. Gait instability in older people with hallux valgus. Foot Ankle Int 2005; 26:483–9.

[11] Menz HB, Morris ME, Lord SR. Footwear characteristics and risk of indoor and outdoor falls in older people. Gerontology 2006;52:174–80.

[12] Menz HB, Tiedemann A, Kwan MM, et al. Foot pain in community-dwelling older people: an evaluation of the Manchester Foot Pain and Disability Index. Rheumatology 2006;45:863–7.

[13] Cooner E, Amorosi S. The study of pain in older Americans. New York: Louis Harris and Associates; 1997.

[14] American Geriatrics Society Panel on Persistent Pain in Older Persons. The management of pain in older persons. J Am Geriatr Soc 2002;50:1–20.

[15] Gibson SJ, Helme RD. Age differences in pain perception and report: a review of physiological, psychological, laboratory, and clinical studies. Pain Reviews 1995;2:65–75.

[16] Helme RD, Gibson SJ. Pain in older people. In: Crombie IK, Croft PR, Linton SJ, et al, editors. Epidemiology of pain. Seattle (WA): IASP Press; 1999. p. 103–12.

[17] Brattberg G, Thorslund M, Wikman A. The prevalence of pain in a general population. The results of a postal survey in a county of Sweden. Pain 1989;37:215–22.

[18] Crook J, Rideout E, Browne G. The prevalence of pain complaints in a general population. Pain 1984;18:299–314.

[19] Magni G, Marchetti M, Moreschi C, et al. Chronic musculoskeletal pain and depressive symptoms in the National Health and Nutrition Examination. Pain 1993;53:163–8.

[20] von Korff M, Dworkin SF, Le Resche L, et al. An epidemiologic comparison of pain complaints. Pain 1988;32:173–83.

[21] Miro J, Paredes S, Rull M, et al. Pain in older adults: a prevalence study in the Mediterranean region of Catalonia. Eur J Pain 2007;11:83–92.

[22] Brochet B, Michel P, Barberger-Gateau P, et al. Population-based study of pain in elderly people: a descriptive survey. Age Ageing 1998;27:279–84.

[23] Roy R, Thomas M. Elderly persons with and without pain: a comparative study. Clin J Pain 1987;3:102–6.

[24] Brattberg G, Parker MG, Thorslund M. The prevalence of pain amongst the oldest old in Sweden. Pain 1996;67:29–34.

[25] Sternbach RA. Survey of pain in the United States: the Nuprin pain report. Clin J Pain 1986; 2:49–53.

[26] Andersson HI, Ejlertsson G, Leden I, et al. Chronic pain in a geographically defined general population: studies of differences in age, gender, social class, and pain localization. Clin J Pain 1993;9:174–82.

[27] Gibson SJ, Helme RD. Age-related differences in pain perception and report. Clin Geriatr Med 2001;17:433–56.

[28] Kendig H, Helme RD, Teshuva K, et al. Health status of older people project: data from a survey of the health and lifestyles of older Australians. Melbourne (Australia): Victorian Health Promotion Foundation; 1996.

[29] Grimby C, Fastbom J, Forsell Y, et al. Musculoskeletal pain and analgesic therapy in a very old population. Arch Gerontol Geriatr 1999;29:29–43.

[30] Jakobsson U, Klevsgard R, Westergren A, et al. Old people in pain: a comparative study. J Pain Symptom Manage 2003;26:625–36.

[31] Helme RD, Gibson SJ. Pain in the elderly. In: Jensen TS, Turner JA, Wiesenfeld-Hallin Z, editors. Proceedings of the 8th World Congress on Pain. Seattle (WA): IASP Press; 1997. p. 919–44.

[32] Jones GT, Macfarlane GJ. Epidemiology of pain in older persons. In: Gibson SJ, Weiner DK, editors. Pain in older persons. Seattle (WA): IASP Press; 2005. p. 3–22.

[33] Paul C, Ayis S, Ebrahim S. Psychological distress, loneliness, and disability in old age. Psychol Health Med 2006;11:221–32.

[34] Cohen-Mansfield J, Parpura-Gill A. Loneliness in older persons: a theoretical model and empirical findings. Int Psychogeriatr 2007;19:279–94.

[35] Wilson RS, Krueger KR, Arnold SE, et al. Loneliness and risk of Alzheimer disease. Arch Gen Psychiatry 2007;64:234–40.

[36] Cacioppo JT, Hughes ME, Waite LJ, et al. Loneliness as a specific risk factor for depressive symptoms: cross-sectional and longitudinal analysis. Psychol Aging 2006;21:140–51.

[37] Hicks TJ Jr. What is your life like now? Loneliness and elderly individuals residing in nursing homes. J Gerontol Nurs 2000;26:15–9.

[38] Sand L, Strang P. Existential loneliness in a palliative home care setting. J Palliat Med 2006; 9:1376–87.

[39] Drageset J. The importance of activities of daily living and social contact for loneliness: a survey among residents in nursing homes. Scand J Caring Sci 2004;18:65–71.

[40] Smitka V. Pain, suffering, and loneliness in the aged. Cas Lek Cesk 1995;134:699–700.

[41] DeWall CN, Baumeister RF. Alone but feeling no pain: effects of social exclusion on physical pain tolerance and pain threshold, affective forecasting, and interpersonal empathy. J Pers Soc Psychol 2006;91:1–15.

[42] Eisenberger NI, Lieberman MD, Williams KD. Does rejection hurt? An FMRI study of social exclusion. Science 2003;302:237–9.

[43] Eisenberger NI, Jarcho JM, Lieberman MD, et al. An experimental study of shared sensitivity to physical pain and social rejection. Pain 2006;126:132–8.

[44] Cole SW, Hawkley LC, Arevalo JM, et al. Social regulation of gene expression in human leukocytes. Genome Biol 2007;8:R189.

[45] Foley DJ, Monjan AA, Brown SL, et al. Sleep complaints among elderly persons: an epidemiologic study of three communities. Sleep 1995;18:425–32.

[46] Ancoli-Israel S, Roth T. Characteristics of insomnia in the United States: results of the 1991 National Sleep Foundations Survey I. Sleep 1999;22:95–103.

[47] Voyer P, Verreault R, Mengue PN, et al. Prevalence of insomnia and its associated factors in elderly long-term care residents. Arch Gerontol Geriatr 2006;42:1–20.

[48] Ohayon MM, Carskadon MA, Guilleminault C, et al. Meta-analysis of quantitative sleep parameters from childhood to old age in healthy individuals: developing normative sleep values across the human lifespan. Sleep 2004;27:1255–73.

[49] Foley D, Ancoli-Israel S, Britz P, et al. Sleep disturbances and chronic disease in older adults: results of the 2003 National Sleep Foundation Sleep in America Survey. J Psychosom Res 2004;56:497–502.

[50] Dick BD, Rashiq S. Disruption of attention and working memory traces in individuals with chronic pain. Anesth Analg 2007;104:1223–9.

[51] Corder LS, Manton KG. National surveys and the health and functioning of the elderly: the effects of design and content. J Am Stat Assoc 1991;86:513–25.

[52] Ives DG, Traven ND, Kuller LH, et al. Selection bias and nonresponse to health promotion in older adults. Epidemiology 1994;5:456–61.

[53] Lord SR, Menz HB. Physiologic, psychologic, and health predictors of 6-minute walk performed in older people. Arch Phys Med Rehabil 2002;83:907–11.

[54] Finucane TE. Overview and critique of the new AGS guideline for management of persistent pain in older adults. Medscape Internal Medicine 2002;4(2):1–6.

[55] Feldt KS. The complexity of managing pain for frail elders. J Am Geriatr Soc 2004;52:840–1.

[56] Chodosh J, Chang JT, Shekelle PG. The quality of medical care provided to vulnerable older patients with chronic pain. J Am Geriatr Soc 2004;52:756–61.

[57] Austrian JS, Kerns RD, Reid MC. Perceived barriers to trying self-management approaches for chronic pain in older persons. J Am Geriatr Soc 2005;53:856–61.

[58] Burgess DJ, van Ryn M, Crowley-Matoka M, et al. Understanding the provider contribution to race/ethnicity disparities in pain treatment: insights from dual process models of stereotyping. Pain Med 2006;7:119–34.

[59] Eich K, Reeves JL, Jaeger B, et al. Memory for pain: relation between past and present pain intensity. Pain 1985;23:375–80.

[60] Jamison RN, Sbrocco T, Parris WCV. The influence of psychosocial factors on accuracy of memory for pain in chronic pain patients. Pain 1989;37:289–94.

[61] Eisenberg DM, Kessler RC, Foster C, et al. Unconventional medicine in the United States. N Engl J Med 1993;328:246–52.

[62] Eisenberg DM, Davis RB, Ettner SL, et al. Trends in alternative medicine use in the United States, 1990–1997: results of a follow-up national survey. JAMA 1998;280:1569–75.

[63] Kessler RC, Davis RB, Foster DF, et al. Long-term trends in the use of complementary and alternative medical therapies in the United States. Ann Intern Med 2001;135:262–8.

[64] Cuellar N, Aycock T, Cahill B, et al. Complementary and alternative medicine (CAM) use by African American (AA) and Caucasian American (CA) older adults in a rural setting: a descriptive, comparative study. BMC Complement Altern Med 2003;3:865.

[65] Flaherty JH, Takahashi R. The use of complementary and alternative medical therapies among older persons around the world. Clin Geriatr Med 2004;20:179–200.

[66] Cuellar NG, Rogers AE, Hisghman V. Evidenc-based research of complementary and alternative medicine (CAM) for sleep in the community-dwelling older adult. Geriatr Nurs 2007;28:46–52.

[67] Tilden VP, Dracg LL, Tolle SW. Complementary and alternative therapy use at end of life in community settings. J Altern Complement Med 2004;10:811–7.

[68] Fleming S, Rabago DP, Mundt MP, et al. CAM therapies among primary care patients using opioid therapy for chronic pain. BMC Complement Altern Med 2007;7:15.

ELSEVIER
SAUNDERS

Clin Geriatr Med 24 (2008) 203–211

CLINICS IN
GERIATRIC
MEDICINE

Pain Perception in the Elderly Patient

Gary McCleane, MD

Rampark Pain Centre, 2 Rampark, Dromore Road, Lurgan,
Northern Ireland BT66 7JH, UK

The challenge of providing pain relief to those who are suffering is often problematic, particularly so in the patient of advanced years. Pain treatment, at its most simple, involves the understanding of what is initiating the pain, how that process can be terminated if possible, and then provision of the most effective pain remedy for that particular type of pain. In reality, things are rarely that simple. It may not be possible to arrest and reverse the causative insult. Regardless of how good any pain-relieving preparation is, it is never effective, or indeed tolerated, in all patients. Then again, pain rarely exists in isolation; thus, cognizance of the patient's condition as a whole has to be taken into account to maximize the chance of effective pain relief being provided. In the elderly patient, these barriers to effective treatment are more substantial. Even the perception of pain may differ from that in those of less advanced years. Of course, many other factors impinge on the presence of, and treatment of, pain in elderly patients, however. Issues of physical accessibility to treatment, cost of drugs, the presence of coexisting illness, the use of concomitant medication, and even the ability to understand the complaints of the patient who has cognitive impairment are only some of those factors that contribute to the complexity of the situation.

Neural changes in the elderly

As with many other organ systems, aging seems to influence morphologic and functional features of the nervous system greatly. In the peripheral nervous system, there is a loss of myelinated and unmyelinated fibers in the elderly, with the decrease in myelin being at least partially attributable to a decrease in expression of the major myelin proteins. Axonal atrophy is also more commonly observed [1]. Nerve conduction and endoneural blood flow are reduced as age advances, and because nerve regeneration is

E-mail address: gary@mccleane.freeserve.co.uk

doi:10.1016/j.cger.2007.12.008
geriatric.theclinics.com

less commonly observed, there may be a reduction in peripheral nerve function [1]. Even when regeneration of damaged neurons occurs, these re-generated fibers have a smaller number of terminal and collateral synapses.

Spinal cord immunochemical studies reveal an increase in mRNA content of the neuropeptide tyrosine and galanin mRNA in dorsal root ganglia (DRG) neurons of aged rats. In these animals, there are decreased cellular contents of calcitonin gene–related peptide (CRGP) and substance P (SP) when compared with younger animals, whereas the levels of somatostatin are similar. The labeling intensity for encoding high-affinity tyrosine receptors (TrkA, TrkB, and TrkC) are decreased in the DRG neurons of aged rats [2].

In addition, there is progressive loss of serotonergic and noradrenergic neurones in the superficial lamina of the spinal dorsal horn [3,4], and be-cause serotonin and norepinephrine have important roles in the descending inhibitory control pathways, such loss may upset the natural endogenous pain-suppressing mechanisms. At supraspinal levels, there is reduced neuro-transmitter content and expression [5]; decreased metabolic turnover; and a loss of neurons and dendritic connections throughout the cerebral cortex, midbrain, and brain stem [6].

Even at the molecular and enzyme levels, changes are seen with aging. For example, the G protein–signaling proteins act as modulators of G protein–coupled receptors, which have a function in opioid signaling. In rats, one such protein, RGS9, is found in increased levels in the caudate-putamen, nucleus accumbens, olfactory tubercle, periaqueductal gray matter, and gray matter of the spinal cord in aged as compared with young animals. In contrast, it is found at decreased levels in the thalamic nuclei and locus coeru-leus in such older animals [7].

It therefore would not seem unreasonable to assume that if there are neural differences between the young and the old, there may also be differences in pain perception and modulation.

Effect of age on results from animal pain models

Some insight into the effect of age on pain perception can be gained from examination of the results of animal pain testing. When nociception is tested in mice using an electrical current, it seems that there are age-related changes in nociception that are curvilinear with the graphic representation of electrical thresholds needed to induce a vocal response being of a U-shaped pattern [8]. That said, not all testing methods definitively show age-related changes, with some being more definitive than others [9,10].

Among those examinations that do reveal age-related changes are those involving SP. It is known that SP levels in the spinal cord of old rats are lower than the levels in young rats. After injury to a peripheral nerve, immu-noreactivity to the SP receptor (neurokinin 1 receptor [NK1]), increases in the spinal cord ipsilateral to the injury and increases the correlation to the development of thermal hyperalgesia. After peripheral nerve injury, aged rats develop thermal hyperalgesia and tactile allodynia more slowly than young rats, and the thermal hyperalgesia correlates with increases in the number of NK1 receptors, with these receptors becoming apparent more slowly [11].

Another animal nociceptive test is that of rat paw incision with measurement of mechanical sensitivity with von Frey filaments and thermal responses assessed with radiant heat. Young and old animals respond in a similar fashion to the thermal stimulus. Younger animals seem to recover more quickly from the mechanical allodynia produced by paw incision when compared with the older animals [12]. This suggests that modulation of A fiber–mediated sensitization differs in young and old rats.

When consideration is given to the formalin test in which formalin application to a paw produces a chronic inflammation characterized by a biphasic response demonstrable by behavioral and electrophysiologic testing, maximum response is seen in middle-aged, as opposed to young or old, animals [13]. An antinociceptive effect in this test is seen when animals are forced to exercise. When mice of varying ages are examined in this variant of the formalin test, the degree of exercise-induced analgesia is maximal in young animals and minimal in the aged animals [14]. This exercise-induced analgesia is not blocked by opioid antagonists but is blocked by N-methyl-D-aspartate receptor antagonists [14].

When we look at isolated neuronal function, studies on spinal cord nociceptive neurons show that spontaneous firing rates are higher and the responses to thermal stimulation are greater in aged as compared with adult rats [15]. Furthermore, the size of the receptive field area of wide dynamic range neurons is larger and that of low-threshold neurons is smaller in aged as compared with adult rats [15]. The increased nociceptive neuronal activity in aged rats correlates with the finding that the paw withdrawal latency is significantly shorter in aged as compared with adult rats after heat stimulation of the paw [12]. This, along with the loss of serotonergic and noradrenergic fibers in the spinal dorsal horn of aged rats [3,4], may contribute to the apparent diminution of descending inhibitory control of nociceptive processing in older animals.

Animal responses to pain stimuli may thus differ when adult and aged animals are examined. Drug effects may differ as well. We are currently seeing increasing use of opioids, particularly "strong" opioids (opioids for severe pain), in the management of chronic pain. Analgesic tolerance is a potential complication of such opioid use. In rat models, tolerance is easy to demonstrate. Wang and colleagues [16] examined rats aged 3 weeks and 3, 6, and 12 months of age. Morphine was injected twice daily, and the time until analgesic tolerance was measured (which they defined as a 75% reduction in morphine-induced analgesia compared with day 1). Tolerance was apparent on days 4, 10, 14, and 22 of morphine treatment. Plasma morphine levels, and levels of its metabolites, did not correlate with the differences in tolerance development.

One other factor that impinges on pain perception is the hormonal status of the patient. We have seen in animal models that advancing age does have a noticeable effect. Particularly in the female animal models, age brings about hormonal changes as well, such that, for example, the response to opioid analgesics is similar in male animals to that of gonadectomized and reproductively senescent female animals but differs from that of reproductively active female animals [17].

Effect of age on human experimental pain

An examination of the effect of age on human experimental pain may give some insight into the clinical relevance of age on pain perception. That said, human experimental pain techniques examine specific modalities of pain, whereas pain is often multimodal in the clinical situation.

There exists a decreased density of myelinated and unmyelinated nerve fibers in older adults with prolonged latencies in peripheral sensory nerves. Older patients may report pain primarily after C-fiber activation, whereas younger adults use additional information from A-δ fibers when reporting pain. When A-δ fiber input was blocked in young adults, age-related differences in pain threshold and differences in subjective ratings of pain intensity disappeared. Cerebral event–related potential (CERP; an electroencephalogram response to any stimulus) in response to noxious stimuli is altered with increasing age, perhaps in part from slowing of the cognitive processing of noxious stimuli and decreased activation of cortical responses in some older adults [18].

Perhaps the most clinically relevant issues are those of pain threshold and pain tolerance. Gibson [19] reports that more than 50 studies have examined age differences in the sensitivity to experimentally induced pain and that most of these studies focus on pain threshold. Twenty-one studies report an increase in pain threshold with advancing age, 3 report a decrease, and 17 report no change. When all results are examined meta-analytically, the effect size is 0.74 ($P<.0005$), indicating that there is definite evidence of an increase in pain threshold with advancing age. If pain tolerance is considered, the 10 studies examining the effect of age on pain tolerance show a definite age-related decrease in the willingness to endure extremely strong pain. The decrease in pain tolerance effect size is estimated at -0.45 ($P<.001$) across these studies [19].

Threshold and tolerance are not the only phenomena that are relevant when pain is considered. For example, Zheng and colleagues [20] studied the effect of age on the response to capsaicin-induced hyperalgesia. Older adults took longer to report first pain, whereas age had no effect on the magnitude of pain reported, flare size, or heat hyperalgesia. This heat hyperalgesia lessened rapidly in all age groups. Punctate hyperalgesia and mechanical pain thresholds remained at higher levels for considerably longer in elderly as opposed to younger adults.

Lasch and colleagues [21] have reported the effect of intraesophageal balloon dilation in healthy young and old adults. The volume of air inflated into the balloon before report of pain was measured. This volume was significantly higher in older subjects. Indeed, many of the older subjects failed to report pain even after maximal balloon inflation, in marked contrast to the younger patients. It certainly seems that when using this experimental technique, pain threshold does increase with age. This study also reminds us that pain is not always an entirely unhelpful symptom, however. On many occasions, it provides a timely warning of impending problems. For example, if it requires a larger volume within a hollow viscus in an elderly patient before pain is experienced as compared with younger subjects, the discomfort caused by an obstructive lesion in the bowel may take longer to become symptomatic in older patients, with all the consequences for the treatment and prognosis of the causative lesion. It is also clinically apparent that the incidence of silent myocardial ischemia increases with age. Whether this is attributable to increased pain threshold in the elderly, a pain-reducing effect of concomitant medication, or the effects of intercurrent illness is debatable, but all may have some effect. Therefore, although our emphasis is on the management of pain in the elderly, we should not lose sight of the fact that thought must also be given to the absence of pain in these patients in circumstances in which it would normally be present.

Along with advancing age comes an increased incidence of such conditions as Alzheimer's disease. Although those with cognitive impairment may have difficulty in communicating the presence of pain, Gibson and colleagues [22] have shown in a model using a heat pain stimulus and subsequent CERP recordings that the presence of Alzheimer's disease did not have any noticeable effect on these pain-evoked potentials when compared with age-matched control subjects. Using a different method of recording evoked potentials, that of auditory-evoked potentials, Harkins [23] has shown that age has no effect on these potentials but that the presence of other sensory impairments, hearing loss in this case, can influence results.

When temporal and spatial summation of pain is considered, it seems that temporal summation to a heat pain stimulus, for example, is more pronounced in the elderly as compared with younger subjects, whereas spatial summation is not significantly influenced by age [24]. One last pain-related phenomenon to consider is that of diffuse noxious inhibitory control, a measure of endogenous pain inhibition. Edwards and colleagues [25] have shown that there is an age-related decrement in diffuse noxious inhibitory control. This may well have an influence on the pain modulatory capacity of elderly subjects.

Effect of age on human clinical pain

Clinical observation would suggest that there is an increased incidence of silent myocardial ischemia in elderly patients, and this exemplifies the fact that advancing age has an effect on pain appreciation. Another example would be the atypical presentation of an inflamed appendix, in which there may be an absence of localized right iliac fossa pain. Differences in the neuroanatomy, physiology, and biochemistry of the nociceptive pathways may cause alterations in pain perception, whereas differences in the pharmacology of drugs in the elderly may alter expected responses to these drugs. Further compounding these issues is the perception of pain in elderly patients by their physicians. Yunis and colleagues [26] compared elderly and young patients who have fibromyalgia. They found that chronic headaches, anxiety, tension, mental stress, and poor sleep were all less common in elderly patients with this condition. Most importantly, however, in only 17% of the elderly patients in the study were the features of fibromyalgia recognized initially by their physician before rheumatologic referral. Many of these patients were exposed to inappropriate corticosteroid treatment in the mistaken belief that they had an inflammatory condition.

The magnitude of the problem of pain in elderly patients is highlighted by figures from Sweden. Here, a survey revealed that 73% of those older than 77 years had pain, whereas 68% of those older than 85 years also had pain [27]. The incidence of pain in the elderly patient is affected by a range of variables, which include racial and ethnic susceptibility to chronic disease, socioeconomic factors, and accessibility to health care [28].

When one tries to consider individual pain conditions, there is a lack of depth of evidence on which to base conclusions. For example, in the case of low back pain, when consideration is given to evidence in published studies, there is a marked underrepresentation of studies that include elderly patients; thus, firm conclusions cannot be reached [29,30]. It is clear, however, that when pain does occur in elderly patients, it has an impact on the overall quality of life of the individual [31]. Analgesic treatment is therefore desirable, remembering that the response of elderly patients to drug therapy may differ from that of younger individuals. It may be that elderly patients require lower dosing of opioid analgesics, have a more rapid response to them, and develop analgesic tolerance more slowly than those of less advanced years [32].

Along with aging comes an increased incidence of such conditions as Alzheimer's disease. It has been observed that the use of nonsteroidal anti-inflammatory drugs is lower in patients who have this condition than in those of a similar age who do not have it and that the use of anti-inflammatories does not depend on the stage of Alzheimer's disease [33]. When patients who have Alzheimer's disease and age-matched controls are again considered, those with acute pain consume a similar quantity of pain killers as those without Alzheimer's disease and it is only in those with chronic pain that consumption is significantly lower [34]. In contrast, patients who have vascular dementia seem to experience more pain than others without cognitive impairment as a result of this condition [35]. In addition to differences in pain experience and analgesic use, cognitive impairment can lead to significant underreporting of pain-related conditions. Indeed, Corali and colleagues [36] found that 41.4% of patients admitted to a geriatric evaluation and rehabilitation unit had previously undiagnosed osteoarthritis.

Overall, therefore, as age advances, the incidence of pain-causing conditions differs from that of younger patients, the impact on quality of life may be greater, and a differing response to analgesic intervention may be observed.

Summary

As with many other health-related issues, the processing, appreciation, and treatment of pain are not uniform during adult life. Neural and biochemical changes accompany aging and may lead to changes in the anatomy and physiology of nociceptive processing. It is becoming clear from experimentation in animal and human models that the consequences of a noxious stimulus differ between young and old subjects.

From a human clinical perspective, therefore, it is of importance to realize how pain and its treatment differ in the elderly patient. Our treatment plans must recognize the alterations in drug pharmacodynamics and pharmacokinetics in older persons and also take into account that there is an increased likelihood of the older patient having concurrent illnesses and taking a variety of medications apart from those with analgesic effects.

Older patients are likely to have an increased pain threshold but to be less tolerant to severe pain. In some circumstances, they may not feel pain when it is appropriate to do so. In other circumstances, pain may be of a different quality or distribution than the pain that one would classically expect. It would be wrong to think of the elderly patient with pain in the same terms as a younger adult from emotional, physiologic, and treatment perspectives.

References

[1] Verdu E, Ceballos D, Vilches JJ, et al. Influence of aging on peripheral nerve function and regeneration. J Peripher Nerv Syst 2000;5:191–208.
[2] Bergman E, Johnson H, Xhang X, et al. Neuropeptides and neurotrophin receptor mRNAs in primary sensory neurons of aged rats. J Comp Neurol 1996;11:303–19.
[3] Wong DF, Wagner HN, Dannals RF. Effects of age on dopamine and serotonin receptors measured by positron tomography in the living human brain. Science 1984;226:1393–6.
[4] Laporte AM, Doyen C, Nevo IT. Autoradiographic mapping of serotonin 5HT1A, 5HT1D, 5HT2A and 5HT3 receptors in the aged human spinal cord. J Chem Neuroanat 1996;11: 67–75.
[5] Barili P, De Carolis G, Zaccheo D, et al. Sensitivity to ageing of the limbic dopaminergic system: a review. Mech Ageing Dev 1998;106:57–92.
[6] Pakkenberg B, Gundersen HJ. Neocortical neuron number in humans: effect of sex and age. J Comp Neurol 1997;384:312–20.
[7] Kim KJ, Moriyama K, Han JB, et al. Differential expression of the regulator of G protein signalling RGS9 protein in nociceptive pathways of different age rats. Brain Res Dev Brain Res 2005;160:28–39.

[8] Finkel JC, Besch VG, Hergen A, et al. Effects of aging on current vocalization threshold in mice measured by a novel nociceptive assay. Anesthesiology 2006;105:360–9.

[9] Gagliese L, Melzack R. Age differences in nonciception and pain behaviour in the rat. Neurosci Biobehav Rev 2000;24:843–54.

[10] Jourdan D, Boghossian S, Alloui A, et al. Age-related changes in nociception and effect of morphine in the Lou rat. Eur J Pain 2000;4:291–300.

[11] Cruce WL, Lovell JA, Crisp T, et al. Effect of aging on the substance P receptor, NK-1, in the spinal cord in rats with peripheral nerve injury. Somatosens Mot Res 2001;18:66–75.

[12] Ririe DG, Vernon TL, Tobin JR, et al. Age dependent responses to thermal hyperalgesia and mechanical allodynia in a rat model of acute postoperative pain. Anesthesiology 2003;99: 443–8.

[13] Gagliese L, Melzack R. Age differences in the response to the formalin test in rats. Neurobiol Aging 1999;20:699–707.

[14] Onodera K, Sakurada S, Furuta S, et al. Age-related differences in forced walking stress-induced analgesia in mice. Drugs Exp Clin Res 2001;27:193–8.

[15] Iwata K, Fukuoda T, Kondo E, et al. Plastic changes in nociceptive transmission of the rat spinal cord with advancing age. J Neurophysiol 2002;10:1086–93.

[16] Wang Y, Mitchell J, Moriyama K, et al. Age-dependent morphine tolerance development in the rat. Anesth Analg 2005;100:1733–9.

[17] Sternberg WF, Ritchie J, Mogil JS. Qualitative sex differences in kappa-opioid analgesia in mice are dependent on age. Neurosci Lett 2004;363:178–81.

[18] Chopra P, Smith H. Acute and chronic pain in the elderly. In: McCleane G, Smith H, editors. Clinical management of the elderly patient in pain. Binghamton (NY): Haworth Press, Inc.; 2006.

[19] Gibson SJ. Pain and aging: the pain experience over the adult lifespan. In: Dostrovsky J, Carr D, Koltzenburg M, editors. Proceedings of the 10th World Congress on Pain. Seattle (WA): IASP Press; 2003.

[20] Zheng Z, Gibson SJ, Khalil Z, et al. Age related differences in the time course of capsaicin induced hyperalgesia. Pain 2000;85:51–8.

[21] Lasch H, Castell DO, Castell JA. Evidence for diminished visceral pain with aging: studies using graded intraesophageal balloon distension. Am J Physiol 1997;272:G1–3.

[22] Gibson SJ, Voukelatos X, Ames D, et al. An examination of pain perception and cerebral-event related potentials following carbon dioxide laser stimulation in patients with Alzheimer's disease and age-matched control volunteers. Pain Res Manag 2001;6:126–32.

[23] Harkins SW. Effects of aged and interstimulus interval on the brainstem auditory evoked potential. Int J Neurosci 1981;15:107–18.

[24] Lautenbacher S, Kunz M, Strate P, et al. Age effects on pain thresholds, temporal summation and spatial summation of heat and pressure pain. Pain 2005;115:410–8.

[25] Edwards RR, Fillingham RB, Ness TJ. Age-related differences in endogenous pain modulation: a comparison of diffuse noxious inhibitory controls in healthy older and younger adults. Pain 2003;101:155–65.

[26] Yunis MB, Holt GS, Masi AT, et al. Fibromyalgia syndrome among the elderly. Comparisons with younger patients. J Am Geriatr Soc 1988;36:987–95.

[27] Brattberg G, Parker MG, Thorslund M. The prevalence of pain among the oldest in Sweden. Pain 1996;67:29–34.

[28] Reyes-Gibby CC, Aday LA, Todd KH, et al. Pain in aging community-dwelling adults in the United States: non-Hispanic whites, non-Hispanic blacks, and Hispanics. J Pain 2007;8: 75–84.

[29] Bressler HB, Keyes WJ, Rochon PA, et al. The prevalence of low back pain in the elderly. A systematic review of the literature. Spine 1999;24:1813–9.

[30] Dionne CE, Dunn KM, Croft PR. Does back pain prevalence really decrease with increasing age? A systematic review. Age Ageing 2006;35:229–34.

[31] Salaffi F, Carotti M, Stancati A, et al. Health-related quality of life in older adults with symptomatic hip and knee osteoarthritis: a comparison with matched healthy controls. Aging Clin Exp Res 2005;17:253–4.

[32] Buntin-Mushock C, Phillip L, Moriyama K, et al. Age-dependent opioid escalation in chronic pain patients. Anesth Analg 2005;100:1740–5.

[33] Scherder EJ, Bouma A. Is decreased use of analgesics in Alzheimer disease due to change in the affective component of pain? Alzheimer Dis Assoc Disord 1997;11:171–4.

[34] Pickering G, Jourdan D, Dubray C. Acute versus chronic pain treatment in Alzheimer's disease. Eur J Pain 2006;10:379–84.

[35] Scherder EJ, Slaets J, Deijen JB, et al. Pain assessment in patients with possible vascular dementia. Psychiatry 2003;66:133–45.

[36] Corali C, Franzoni S, Gatti S, et al. Diagnosis of chronic pain caused by osteoarthritis and prescription of analgesics in patients with cognitive impairment. J Am Med Dir Assoc 2006; 7:1–5.

ELSEVIER
SAUNDERS

Clin Geriatr Med 24 (2008) 213–236

CLINICS IN
GERIATRIC
MEDICINE

Assessment of Pain in the Elderly Adult

Patricia Bruckenthal, PhD, RN, ANP-BC[a,b,*]

[a]Department of Adult and Family Health Nursing, School of Nursing,
Stony Brook University, HSC, L2, Room 224, Stony Brook, NY 11794–8240, USA
[b]Pain and Headache Treatment Center,
North Shore/Long Island Jewish Health System, Department of Neurology,
1554 Northern Boulevard, 4th Floor, Manhassett, NY 11030, USA

The goals of a clinical assessment for pain in the elderly adult may be similar to those established for younger patients; however, unique characteristics of aging make this assessment more challenging for clinicians. These characteristics include reluctance of older individuals to report pain; the assumption that pain is a normal part of aging; sensory and cognitive impairments; and fear of the consequences of acknowledging pain, such as expensive testing or hospitalization. In addition, older adults often have multiple comorbidities that impact on the pain presentation. The pain experience can influence mood, physical functioning, and social interactions, and indicates that pain assessment in older adults is a multidimensional and often multidisciplinary responsibility.

The overarching goal of pain assessment in the elderly is to provide successful pain management. This is predicated on a successful and comprehensive pain assessment. Specific goals include (1) determining the presence and cause of pain; (2) identifying exacerbating comorbidities; (3) reviewing beliefs, attitudes, and expectations regarding pain; and (4) gathering information that assists and impacts an individualized treatment plan [1]. Ultimately, this assessment yields a treatment plan that results in positive outcomes including decreased pain and increased function and quality of life.

This article provides the clinician with the foundation to perform a successful pain assessment for older adults who are able to communicate by self-report. This provides a comprehensive base on which to build a relevant plan of care. Pain assessment for those with cognitive impairment is the focus of the article by Bjoro and Herr elsewhere in this issue.

* HSC, Level 2, Room 224, Stony Brook, NY 11794–8240.
  E-mail address: patricia.bruckenthal@stonybrook.edu

0749-0690/08/$ - see front matter © 2008 Elsevier Inc. All rights reserved.
doi:10.1016/j.cger.2007.12.002

Prevalence of pain in older adults

Prevalence statistics for persistent pain in older adults range from 25% to 80%. Pain prevalence reports vary depending on whether the older adults reside in a nursing home (45%–80% Refs. [2,3]) or are community dwelling (25%–50% Refs. [4,5]). Pain continues to be an underassessed and undertreated condition in this population [6,7].

Lack of familiarity of common age-related changes and common painful conditions among the elderly may contribute to the underrecognition of the problem. Many times diagnostic imaging studies are poorly correlated with the clinical expressions of pain. This may lead to confusion on the part of the examining clinician and the potential for undervaluing the self-report of the patient and poor treatment planning. A list of pain syndromes common in older adults is outlined in Box 1.

Musculoskeletal pain is one of the most common types of pain experienced by community-dwelling older adults [8–10]. The underlying disorders responsible for chronic low back pain are varied and require specific physical examination techniques. For example, of 111 older adults with chronic low back pain, 84% reported sacroiliac joint pain, 19% reported pain consistent with fibromyalgia, 96% reported myofacial pain, and 48% reported hip pain [11]. Rheumatic diseases, characterized by inflammation,

---

Box 1. Common pain syndromes in older adults

Musculoskeletal conditions
 Osteoarthritis
 Degenerative disk disease
 Osteoporosis and fractures
 Gout

Neuropathic conditions
 Diabetic neuropathy
 Postherpatic neuralgia
 Trigeminal neuralgia
 Central poststroke pain
 Radicular pain secondary to degenerative disease of the spine

Rheumatologic conditions
 Rheumatoid arthritis
 Polymyalgia rheumatica
 Fibromyalgia

Data from Hadjistavropoulos T, Herr K, Turk DC, et al. An interdisciplinary expert consensus statement on assessment of pain in older persons. Clin J Pain 2007;23(Suppl 1):S1–43; and Hanks-Bell M, Halvey K, Paice JA. Pain assessment and management in aging. Online J Issues Nurs 2004;9(3):8.

degeneration, or metabolic disorders, are the most common disease reported by older adults residing in long-term care facilities [12]. Specific examination techniques for musculoskeletal disorders are discussed later.

Functional, cognitive, emotional, and societal consequences have been associated with unrelieved pain in older adults. Decreased activity because of pain can lead to myofacial deconditioning and gait disturbances, which in turn can result in injuries from falls. Appetite impairment has been reported in community-dwelling adults with pain intensity scores higher than those without appetite impairment [13]. Pain in the elderly has been associated with increased sleep disturbances [14]. These consequences can lead to less than optimal participation in rehabilitation efforts and decreased quality of life in general. Increased costs because of health care use have also been implicated as a result of unrelieved pain in the elderly [15]. Consideration of the unique characteristics included in the history and physical assessment for pain in older adults' assists clinicians in the development and implementation of an individualized treatment plan that optimizes successful outcomes.

Elements of a comprehensive assessment

A comprehensive, multidimensional pain assessment in older adults ultimately leads to a more successful individualized plan of care. Regardless of whether the pain is acute, postoperative, or chronic, the goal of the assessment is to identify the cause of pain, conduct a thorough history of comorbid medical and psychosocial conditions, and perform an appropriate physical examination and diagnostic work-up. Often a multidisciplinary approach may be needed, and after the initial assessment, the clinician may determine that referral to an appropriate specialist is necessary for specialized services or skilled procedures. For example, a mental health professional may be able to optimize a plan to treat depression or a substance abuse disorder, or a physical therapist may be consulted for evaluation of a conditioning program. A review of existing medical records is also beneficial in the assessment process.

History of the pain complaint

There are several elements recognized as essential for a comprehensive assessment of pain at any age. One such schema recommended for guiding a comprehensive pain assessment in older adults is outlined in detail in the Initiative on Methods, Measurement, and Pain Assessment in Clinical Trials project [1,16–18]. Included in this review are necessary elements including nuances specific to older adults to assist the clinician in the assessment process. Techniques for assessing these age-specific elements are included below.

Self-report of pain is still considered the most reliable source for the cognitively intact and communicative older adult's pain complaint [19]. Sensory deficits in vision, hearing, and cognition are common in this population and need to be identified before beginning the interview. These may impact on the patient's ability to complete the assessment process and adjustments to accommodate for deficits need to be considered. This may become especially relevant when selecting appropriate pain assessment instruments. It also may be beneficial to query other family members or caregivers for additional perspective on medical history, predominant mood and affect, and physical and social functioning.

Present pain complaint

Assessment of the pain characteristics includes a detailed description of the onset, duration, frequency, intensity, location, and contributing factors. For a variety of reasons older adults may not be forthcoming regarding reports of pain. They also may use description other than pain to describe what they are experiencing. It is common for older adults to use such terms as "aching," "soreness," "hurting," "discomfort" [20,21], or other descriptors.

The onset and timing are important considerations. Although degenerative musculoskeletal disorders generally have an insidious onset, a change in character from a less severe to a more intense pain may indicate a progression of disease or a new-onset fracture. Pain that is more intense in the morning is a feature of cancerous bone pain. Tools to evaluate pain intensity specific to the geriatric population have been identified and are outlined later. Older persons are able to use a body pain map or diagram to indicate the locations of their pain [22,23]. Sometimes the pain, although not present during rest, manifests itself during activities and this too should be explored with the patient. A useful structured interview technique that elicits information on the present pain complaint for older adults who can communicate is suggested in Box 2. Associated symptoms, such as paresthesias, may indicate radicular involvement of an extremity in pain. Fever or weight loss may herald more ominous diagnoses including infection or malignancy.

Past medical history

This review should include a history of past medical, surgical, and psychiatric conditions, and accidents or injuries. Dates of onset, current and past treatments, and treating practitioners should be obtained. Eliciting this information is important for several reasons. The existence of certain comorbid conditions impacts treatment decisions for pain. For example, nonsteroidal anti-inflammatory agents may be limited in those with a history of heart disease or hypertension. Patients with liver disease need to use acetaminophen cautiously. Pre-existing renal disease also affects the use of medications. Identification and documentation of pre-existing conditions facilitates treatment planning.

Box 2. Assessment of brief pain impact for verbal patients

1. How strong is your pain (right now, worst or average over past week)?
2. How many days over the past week have you been unable to do what you would like to do because of your pain?
3. Over the past week, how often has pain interfered with your ability to take care of yourself, for example with bathing, eating, dressing, and going to the toilet?
4. Over the past week, how often has pain interfered with your ability to take care of your home-related chores, such as going grocery shopping, preparing meals, paying bills, and driving?
5. How often do you participate in pleasurable activities, such as hobbies, socializing with friends, and travel? Over the past week, how often has pain interfered with these activities?
6. How often do you do some sort of exercise? Over the past week, how often has pain interfered with your ability to exercise?
7. Does pain interfere with your ability to think clearly?
8. Does pain interfere with your appetite? Have you lost weight?
9. Does pain interfere with your sleep? How often over the past week?
10. Has pain interfered with your energy, mood, personality, or relationship with other people?
11. Over the past week, how often have you taken pain medications?
12. How would you rate your health at the present time?

From Weiner D, Herr K. Comprehensive interdisciplinary assessment and treatment planning: an integrative overview. In: Weiner D, Herr K, Rudy T, editors. Persistent pain in older adults: an interdisciplinary guide for treatment. New York: Springer; 2002. p. 18–57; with permission.

Knowledge of the pattern of certain pre-existing conditions can also help with anticipatory planning. Sensory distal polyneuropathy is the most common neurologic presentation in patients with diabetes mellitus. Although most are painless, 7.5% report unpleasant sensations of pain [24]. Clinicians should be alert to evolving sensory complaints in diabetic patients, especially those with poor glycemic control. Musculoskeletal disorders that have changed in presentation may signal progression of disease and may require more intense investigation. Finally, results of any previous laboratory and diagnostic tests should be reviewed not only to guide future treatment decisions, but to avoid unnecessary repeat testing.

Medication history

A careful medication history must be inclusive of all current and past medications, dosages, side effects, and response. This consists of prescribed, over-the-counter, and herbal supplements. Alcohol use should be specific to frequency and amount. Tobacco products and illicit drug use are also important elements of inquiry. It is important to obtain the name and telephone number of the current pharmacy used.

Functional assessment

Essential elements of a functional assessment are broad and include cognitive, physical, and psychosocial dimensions. Data from these aspects of the assessment establish a baseline to enable the clinician to determine specific goals, the extent to which the patient can participate, and response to the treatment plan.

Cognition is grossly assessed during the process of the health interview. Some areas of cognitive decline, such as fluid reasoning, processing speed, and short-term memory, are part of the normal aging process [25,26]. Factors other than dementia that should be considered as causative factors in cognitive decline include poor nutritional status, medication effect, depression, living environment [25], and pain [27]. The Mini Mental State Exam [28] can be used to assess cognition, but may not be able to pick up subtle changes. A more complete discussion on pain assessment in the cognitively impaired adult is addressed in the article by Herr, elsewhere in this issue.

Physical function incorporates the assessment of mobility, activities of daily living, sleep pattern, and appetite. The clinician should ascertain the current level of physical activity and mobility of which the patient is capable. This includes assessment of the level basic activities of daily living are being performed. It is helpful to identify activities previously performed that the pain prohibits the patient from doing currently. Ask if the patient engages in a regular exercise program. These assessment parameters should establish the baseline of current physical function.

Questions regarding sleep patterns are asked to evaluate if restorative sleep is being attained. Poor sleep may be the result of the aging process, depression, or pain. Identifying the cause assists in developing an appropriate intervention for improving sleep. Appetite suppression has been associated with higher pain intensity level in community-dwelling adults [13]. Poor nutrition can contribute to fatigue and diminished function and well-being. By reviewing all the pertinent aspects of function, the clinician and patients can begin to establish realistic treatment goals in this domain.

Psychosocial assessment

Mood, social support systems, recreational involvement, and financial resources are important to the psychosocial assessment. These factors all influence the pain experience and how the patient in pain functions in these domains and responds to various treatments.

Depressive disorders are prevalent in people with chronic pain [14,29–31]. Patients who are depressed may exhibit decreased energy, engagement in treatment modalities, or avoidance of pleasant diversional activities. The Geriatric Depression Scale [32] is one instrument that can be used to determine if further evaluation for depression is indicated. This instrument is of particular benefit in residential care elders, whereas the Center for Epidemiological Studies Depression Scale [33,34] is more suited for community-dwelling elders [35].

Anxiety has also been closely associated with pain [36,37] and often coexists with depression in this population. Anxiety may play a part in fear-related behavior that might inhibit participation in physical rehabilitation efforts. It may be useful for the clinician under these circumstances to evaluate this disorder in more detail. The Beck Anxiety Inventory [38] is a brief screen tool that has been used in the elderly for evaluating anxiety symptoms. A distinction can be made between a situational anxiety response and the more enduring personality anxiety trait and evaluated using the State-Trait Anxiety Inventory [39]. Although eliciting trait versus state anxiety traits, it may be noted in pain patients, the relationship between transient and enduring emotional responses to pain and outcomes to treatment intervention need to be further explored. Emotional responses of depression and anxiety, however, do have an impact on the overall pain experience and are essential to the overall assessment.

Assessment of the social support network and economic status for older people in pain is important on several levels. Involvement with family and friends can provide pleasurable experiences and diversion away from a constant focus on pain. Supportive social contacts can provide transportation to clinic and treatment appointments. Osteoarthritis patients who participated in spouse-assisted pain-coping skills training had greater reduction on pain and disability outcomes that those who participated in conventional nonspousal participant training [40]. In addition to the availability of social support, the type of relationship should be assessed. Negative social reinforcement may present in the form of overly solicitous family members who encourage sedentary behavior. Other negative effects are likely if long-term caregivers become resentful of their support role. Finally, economic resources have a great impact on access to potential treatment options and must be identified.

Beliefs and attitudes about pain

The context in which older adults perceive pain is relevant to the overall assessment. Pain can signify loss of independence, debilitating illness, or be regarded as a general consequence of the aging process and underreported. Better treatment satisfaction and outcomes are reported when there is greater agreement between patients' beliefs about the nature and treatment of pain and the treatment received [41].

Multiple constructs associated with beliefs and attitudes about pain have been studied and have an impact on the total pain experience and outcomes. Many of these are interrelated, such as coping, self-efficacy, catastrophizing, and pain-related fears. Coping and self-efficacy are discussed later.

Two simplistic models of coping have been described as active versus passive [42–44] and adaptive versus maladaptive coping [45,46]. Patients use a variety of coping skills for managing pain. For example, task persistence, activity pacing, and use of coping self-statements were coping strategies most frequently used by a group of predominately female older adults living in retirement facilities [47]. Prayer is often used by older adult women as a coping mechanism for pain [48]. Identifying coping skills among the elderly is important so that the clinician can encourage the use of previously successful skills or modify treatment interventions to incorporate teaching effective coping skills. Patients with passive or maladaptive coping styles likely benefit from psychologic interventions [49] that focus on more effective ways of coping.

Self-efficacy refers to the belief that one can control or manage certain outcomes of one's life [50,51]. Beliefs about the degree of control and self-efficacy in being able to manage pain have been well studied [52,53] and are related to types of coping strategies used to manage pain [54]. Participation in cognitive-behavioral pain-coping skills interventions can increase self-efficacy beliefs and have been shown to decrease pain intensity, disability, and depression [40,55–57]. Patients who are identified as having poor beliefs regarding their ability to manage pain may benefit from coping skills training aimed at increasing self-efficacy. Examples of instruments that measure one's perceived ability to manage pain are listed in Table 1.

Pain assessment measurement instruments

There are an abundance of reliable and valid instruments available to assist in the assessment of pain. The choice of which to use depends on factors including purpose of the tool, clinical setting, and time constraints. Some instruments measure a single pain construct, whereas others are multidimensional. Clinicians are encouraged to find instruments that are useful to their clinical needs and encompass the broad pain assessment domains covered in this article.

Table 1 represents a sample of pain assessment instruments that were extrapolated from reviews by Hadjistavropoulos and colleagues, Gibson and Weiner, and Herr and Garand. Many of these are self-assessment and self-report instruments and can be administered before the history and examination portion of the pain assessment and reviewed by the clinician with the patient. The choice of tools can be overwhelming. As a pragmatic yet comprehensive approach, Hadjistavropoulos and colleagues [1] recommends the administration of the Brief Pain Inventory [58] and the Short Form McGill Pain Questionnaire [59] as suitable for most cognitively intact older adults. These cover the multidimensional nature of the pain assessment and can be completed in approximately 10 minutes. Instruments that measure pain in cognitively impaired elders are covered in the article by Bjoro and Herr elsewhere in this issue.

Physical assessment

General

The focus of the physical assessment varies depending on whether the pain complaint is acute or chronic. In general, inflammation, traumatic injury, and cancer-related conditions are associated with acute pain, whereas neurologic and musculoskeletal etiologies cause more chronic pain conditions. This section focuses on the latter assessment and suggestions for the former are included in the discussion of assessment of specific painful conditions. All patients should have a brief examination of general health status including vision and hearing, cardiovascular, respiratory, and gastrointestinal systems before the more focused examination.

When examining the painful region inspection is focused on signs of inflammation; trophic changes; joint deformity; and vascular signs, such as paleness, cyanosis, or mottled appearance.

Musculoskeletal examination

Assessment of the musculoskeletal system focuses on inspection of any joint deformities and disuse signs, such as asymmetry of muscular bulk and tone. Note any spinal deformity including kyphosis, lordosis, or scoliosis. Palpation includes the spinous processes and paraspinal muscles, sacroiliac joint, piriformis, or the fibromyalgia tender points for more generalized pain complaints. During range of motion of the cervical spine, lumbar spine, and hip, the quality, quantity, and elicitation of pain should be noted.

Specific examination maneuvers can offer clues to the etiology of the pain complaint. Straight leg raising (Lasègue's sign) is indicative of nerve root compression. Crossed straight leg raising (exacerbation of leg pain when the contralateral leg is raised) may suggest lumbar disk herniation, but may also occur with sacroiliac pathology. Fabere maneuvers (Patrick's test) include flexion, extension, abduction, and external rotation of the hip. Pain during these movements is suggestive of degenerative joint disease of the hip. Pain radiating down the arm produced by lateral tilt or rotation of the head (Spurling's sign) in patients complaining of neck pain may indicate cervical nerve root compression. Lhermitte's sign is an electric shock–like sensation in the torso or extremities associated with cervical flexion and may be suggestive of a cervical cord lesion [60].

Mobility and balance

Pain is a contributing factor of mobility impairment and falls in the elderly and warrants an assessment of gait and balance. Gait changes

Table 1
Selected instruments for pain assessment in older adults

Domain	Instrument	Instrument characteristics	Psychometrics established by setting	Comments
Pain intensity	Numeric Rating Scale	Available in a variety of scale ranges including 0–5, 0–10, 0–20, and 0–100	Acute care Subacute care Pain clinic Long-term care Assisted living Community dwelling	Preferred by many older adults Verbal version may be difficult for elders with cognitive impairment Vertical orientation of scale easier to use for elders
	Verbal Descriptor Scale	Available in a variety of scale types including: 5-point verbal rating scale Pain thermometer [75] Present pain inventory [76] Graphic rating scale [77]	Acute care Subacute care Pain clinic Long-term care Assisted living Community dwelling	Most preferred by older adults Requires abstract thought Thermometer adaptation may assist with tool understanding [78]
	Pictorial Pain Scales	Facial pain scales tested in older adults: Faces Pain Scale [79] Wong-Baker FACES Scale [80]	Acute care Subacute care Pain clinic Long-term care Assisted living Community dwelling Community dwelling	Preferred by many older adults Validated in white, African American, and Spanish Does not require language Required abstract thinking
Multidimensional pain assessment	Short Form McGill Pain Questionnaire [59]	15 pain quality words rated on a Likert scale, plus a VAS of pain intensity, plus a present pain inventory	Community dwelling Pain clinic Acute care	Measures sensory and affective dimensions Not recommended for illiterate or cognitively impaired

Instrument	Description	Setting	Comments
Brief Pain Inventory [58]	11-item instrument that gathers information on pain severity and level of pain interference on seven key aspects of function	Multiple settings including cancer, chronic pain conditions, postoperative pain, and older adults	Measures intensity and pain interference; Does not measure quality or affective dimensions of pain; Available in over 30 languages
Pain Disability Index [81]	7 items using 11-point scale to measure perceived pain interference with the performance of seven areas of daily function	Community dwelling; Chronic pain	Measures pain-related disability; Short and easy to use; Needs further study for use in outcomes measures
Geriatric Pain Measure [82]	24-item questionnaire measuring five clusters of components: pain intensity, disengagement, pain with ambulation, pain with strenuous activities, and pain with other activities	Ambulatory geriatric clinic	Measures intensity, interference, disengagement, and pain with activity; Limited evaluation data
Multidimensional Pain Inventory [83]	61-item, comprised of 13 subscales across three sections	Multiple settings; Pain clinic	Measures pain intensity, interference, significant other support, general activity; Cross culturally validated; Identifies adaptation styles and response to treatment; Lengthy to complete, approximately 20 min; Limited psychometric study in the elderly
Functional Pain Scale [84]	0–5 scored tool that combines pain severity and function and rates ability to tolerate activity	Community dwelling	Measures intensity and function; Limited by indicators that measure interference based on ability to watch TV, read, and use a telephone

(continued on next page)

Table 1 (continued)

Domain	Instrument	Instrument characteristics	Psychometrics established by setting	Comments
Functional status	Functional Status Index [85]	Two self-administered subscales; pain and difficulty. Difficulty subscale focuses attention on task performance rather than amount of pain experienced while performing the task	Acute care	Measures basic ADL and instrumental ADL. Takes approximately 8 min to administer
	Physical Activity Scale [86]	Measures levels of physical activity in past week in areas of leisure, occupation, and household activities	Community dwelling	Measures basic, instrumental, and advanced ADL. 8 min to complete
Site-specific disability	Oswestry Disability Scale [87]	10 items measuring level of pain and interference with physical activities, sleep, self-care, sex life, social life, and travel	Primary care	Evaluates low back pain. Measures basic, instrumental, and advanced ADL. 5 min to complete
	Rowland Morris Disability Index [75]	24-item instrument derived from the Sickness Impact Profile where the phrase "because of my back" was added to each statement, making it disease specific	Included, but not specific to older adults	Evaluates low back pain. Measures basic and instrumental ADL. 5 min to complete
	Western Ontario and McMaster Universities Osteoarthritis Index [88]	24-item instrument that assesses pain, disability, and joint stiffness	Included, but not specific to older adults	Evaluates hip and knee pain. 8 min to complete
	Neck Pain and Disability Index [89]	20-item instrument designed to measure intensity of pain and interference with vocational, recreational, social, and self-care activities and emotions	Included, but not specific to older adults	Evaluates neck pain. 5 min to complete

Cognitive processes; pain specific			
Cognitive Errors Questionnaire [90]	48 vignettes assessing four depression-related cognitive disorders: catastrophizing, overgeneralization, personalization, and selective abstraction. Half of the vignettes use chronic pain as the stimulus for the situation	Adults with rheumatoid arthritis, including but not specific to older adults	
Inventory of Negative Thoughts in Response to Pain [91]	21 five-point items comprising three subscales: negative self-statements, negative social cognitions, and self-blame	Included, but not specific to older adults	
Pain Attitudes Questionnaire [92]	27 items load on four factors representing stoicism (superiority, reticence) and cautiousness (self-doubt, reluctance)	Community dwelling	Age-related increase in degree of reticence to pain, self-doubt, and reluctance to label a sensation as painful was found
Pain Catastrophizing Scale [93]	13 items comprise three subscales describing catastrophizing thinking: helplessness, rumination, and magnification	Not known	
Arthritis Helplessness Index [94]	5 items tapping perceived uncontrollability of arthritis symptoms	Included, but not specific to older adults	Helplessness correlated with greater age, lesser education, lower self-esteem, lower internal health locus of control, higher anxiety, and depression, and impairment in performing ADL
Arthritis self-efficacy Scale [95]	20 items measuring self-efficacy in three domains: pain, function, and other symptoms	Primary care Community dwelling	Health outcomes and self-efficacy scores improved when patients participated in the Arthritis Self-Management Course

(continued on next page)

Table 1 (*continued*)

Domain	Instrument	Instrument characteristics	Psychometrics established by setting	Comments
Affective processes	Pain Anxiety Symptoms Scale [96]	62 items comprising four subscales: fear of pain, cognitive anxiety, somatic anxiety, escape and avoidance	Multidisciplinary pain clinic Included, but not specific to older adults	May be useful in the continued study of fear of pain and its contribution to the development and maintenance of pain behaviors
	Beck Anxiety Inventory [38]	21 items answered on a four-point scale		
	Tampa Scale of Kinesiophobia [97]	17 items addressing fears about pain and reinjury	Not known	For older chronic pain patients, a stronger mediating role for pain-related fear was supported [98]
				Items may represent catastrophic thinking, rather than fear of movement [99]
	Survey of Activities and Fear of Falling in the Elderly [100]	11 items, subscales include activity, restriction, fear of falling, and activity level		May be able to differentiate fear of falling that leads to activity restriction from fear of falling that accompanies activity
	Geriatric Depression Scale [32]	30 yes/no items; omits somatic and other depressive symptoms possible confounded with aging	Community dwelling Long-term care facility	Short form available Performed better than the Center for Epidemiological Studies Depression Scale in residential settings for elders
	Center for Epidemiological Studies Depression Scale [33]	20 four-point items	Community dwelling Long-term care facility	Performed better than the Geriatric Depression Scale in community-dwelling elders

Coping skills	Coping Strategies Questionnaire [101]	42 items assess seven strategies (making coping self-statements, ignoring pain sensations, reinterpreting pain sensations, praying and hoping, catastrophizing, diverting attention, and increasing activities) but various factor structures have emerged		Widely used in older adults, especially those with osteoarthritis
	Chronic Pain Coping Inventory [102]	65 items assess behavioral coping strategies in 11 domains		Short form available Has been used, but not validated in older adults
	Vanderbilt Pain Management Inventory [42]	Separate active (11 items) and passive (7 items) subscales		
	Coping with Chronic Illness [103,104]	54 items comprise six subscales: cognitive restructuring, emotional expression, wishfullfilling fantasy, self blame, information seeking, and threat minimizing	Included, but not specific to older adults	Not pain specific
	Ways of Coping Scale (Revised) [105]	66 items comprise numerous subscales and two higher-order factors: problem-focused and emotion-focused coping; revised		Not pain specific

Abbreviation: ADL, activities of daily living.

Data from Hadjistavropoulos T, Herr K, Turk DC, et al. An interdisciplinary expert consensus statement on assessment of pain in older persons. Clin J Pain 2007;23(Suppl 1):S1–43; Gibson SJ, Weiner DK. Pain in older persons. Seattle (WA): IASP Press; 2005; Herr KA, Garand L. Assessment and measurement of pain in older adults. Clin Geriatr Med 2001;17:457–78.

associated with aging include decreased step length, walking speed, ankle range of motion, and the ability to push-off with the toes. The ability to rise unassisted from a seated position to standing, timed and averaged for five repetitions [61], and the "timed up and go" tests [62] are simple, quick measures of basic functional mobility.

Neurologic

When conducting a focused neurologic examination, strength, sensation, and deep tendon reflexes are assessed. In general, a sensory dermatomal level usually correlates with the anatomic level of the lesion. Hyperalgesia, hyperpathia, and hypoesthesia can be tested by pinprick. Allodynia is tested using a cotton swab or paint brush. Hyporeflexia may indicate nerve root compression, whereas hyperreflexia may be indicative of myelopathy from spinal cord compression. Decreased vibratory sensation and hyporeflexia are signs consistent with peripheral neuropathy.

The physical assessment is important to help confirm etiology and identify level of impairment, to determine level of function, and to elicit emergent conditions in the older population. Ongoing physical assessment continues to be imperative to evaluate the effectiveness of treatment, exacerbation of identified conditions, or the emergence of new problems that need attention. A follow-up physical examination guided by the medical history should take place at each subsequent visit.

Assessment considerations for specific painful conditions

Trigeminal neuralgia

Trigeminal neuralgia is characterized by severe, unilateral facial pain described as lancinating electric shock–like jolts in one or more distributions of the trigeminal nerve. The maxillary and mandibular divisions are most commonly affected. The causes vary by age. In the elderly, compression of the trigeminal root by an artery or vein or both is the cause about 80% of the time. Intracranial tumors and demyelinating disease have also been implicated. The characteristic jabs of pain last from 2 to 120 seconds and are often precipitated by such activities as brushing, chewing, or talking. The paroxysms of pain are separated by pain-free intervals. Because there are no cranial nerve deficits, the diagnosis of tumor may be delayed. Careful clinical evaluation and MRI is recommended for all patients presenting with trigeminal neuralgia [63].

Postherpetic neuralgia

Postherpetic neuralgia is a frequent complication following an outbreak of herpes zoster in the elderly. Sensory findings include allodynia or hyperalgesia in the associated dermatomal region, the thoracic being more common than the facial. Patients with allodynia complain of the wind or a piece of clothing causing pain. Hyperalgesic patients describe provocation of pain by a relatively mild stimulus, such as bumping up against a piece of furniture. Tingling, severe itching, burning, or steady throbbing pain has also been described. Pain associated with postherpetic neuralgia can interfere with activities of daily living and quality of life; identification and intervention is crucial [63].

Poststroke pain

Poststroke pain, an underrecognized consequence following stroke, occurs in 33% to 40% of patients who have had a stroke. The pain may present as shoulder pain in the paretic limb or present as central poststroke pain. Central poststroke pain is characterized as pain that is severe and persistent with accompanying sensory abnormalities [64,65].

Metastatic bone pain

Bone pain that is worse at night, when lying down, or not associated with acute injury should raise suspicion of metastatic disease. Also, pains that gradually but rapidly increase in intensity or with weight-bearing or activity are suspicious. Frequent sites of metastatic pain include the hip, vertebrae, femur, ribs, and skull. Examination includes palpation of the affected site.

Temporal arteritis

Greater than 95% of the cases of temporal arteritis occur in patients over 50 years old. Presentation includes complaints of new-onset headache, malaise, scalp tenderness, and jaw claudication. Physical examination reveals an indurated temporal artery that is tender with a diminished or absent pulse. Because irreversible blindness is a consequence if untreated, timely assessment and treatment is essential [66]. Generally, patients are started on glucocorticoids while awaiting temporal artery biopsy.

Setting of the pain assessment

Much of the current literature on pain assessment and information provided in this article seem most suited for elders with chronic pain rather that acute pain. Psychosocial factors are more closely associated with chronic pain states and have been studied more intensely. The nature of the pain being evaluated and setting of evaluation dictate which assessment techniques are warranted. Although scales that measure pain intensity can be administered rapidly and are suitable for any setting, others require more time and are more likely to be helpful in the primary care office or clinic or long-term care facility. Some distinctions regarding the setting and type of pain are provided next.

Acute pain

Older adults who present with acute pain require a rapid assessment in-cluding a self-report of pain intensity, and other descriptors of the present pain complaint. Past pain history and medication history are also essential. Completion of a more comprehensive assessment can be delayed until the etiology and treatment of the pain has been initiated. Ongoing monitoring of the pain intensity, duration, and effects of treatment should take place every 2 to 4 hours initially. Once every 8 hours is appropriate once the pain is well controlled [67].

Older hospitalized acute pain patients were reported to use fewer descrip-tors to describe pain than chronic pain patients in a hospital rehabilitation unit. Acute pain patients used "piercing and burning" to describe pain, whereas "piercing, pulling, spreading, and shooting" were frequently used by patients in chronic pain [68]. Older adults may use terms other than pain, so questions that ask about discomfort and hurting may need to be asked [20]. The patient should be observed during an activity, such as ambulation, transfers, or repositioning, because behavior and pain levels may not be equal during different activities [20].

Autonomic responses, such as increased heart rate and blood pressure and altered respiratory rate, are generally associated with acute pain. The clinician should be cautioned that the absence of these signs does not indi-cate that pain is not present [69]. No statistically significant differences were seen between self-reported pain scores and heart rate, blood pressure, or respiratory rate in adult patients presenting to an emergency department for a variety of acute painful conditions [70]. Clinicians should not rely on vital signs as the sole indicator for the presence or degree of acute pain. Patient self-report of pain remains the gold standard.

Long-term care facility

Pain assessment in nursing homes continues to be a challenge. Common themes regarding pain assessment in long-term care facilities persist. Two recent studies illustrate the significance of this problem.

Clark and colleagues [71] conducted a qualitative study using focus groups in 12 nursing homes in Colorado. They identified that within nursing homes (1) there is an uncertainty in pain assessment; (2) that relationship-centered cues to residents' pain is a solution to limitations of formal assess-ment; (3) cues to pain are behavioral changes and observable physical changes; and (4) specific residents' characteristics, such as attitudes or being perceived as difficult, made pain assessment more challenging. These find-ings have implications for practice. Education of staff regarding the complex nature of chronic pain and its' psychosocial domains may help clarify the ambiguity expressed regarding assessment. Acknowledging the importance of family members and certified nursing assistants' reports of behavioral and physical changes is essential to the process. The use of pain assessment tools appropriate for "difficult" patients or patients with communication impairment is helpful. It has been reported that the availability of various assessment tools to suit patient preferences increases the frequency of diagnosing pain in nursing home residents [72].

Similarly, Kaasalainen and colleagues [73] found that pain assessment was problematic in nursing homes and that appropriate pain assessment strategies were closely linked to effective pain management. Common themes of negative myths about pain and aging, inadequacy of current tools used in practice, and the inability to discriminate between pain and such problems as dementia and delirium emerged. This lack of confidence in assessment was reflected in the ways that pain was treated.

These findings suggest that engaging in a process committed to pain assessment at all levels in the long-term care facility has positive implications for management of pain in this setting. Two useful resources to facilitate implementing an institutional plan are described in the American Geriatric Society Panel on Persistent Pain in Older Adults [19] and the American Medical Directors Association Chronic Pain Management in the Long Term Care Setting guidelines [74]. These are evidence-based interdisciplinary guidelines that form a basis for a comprehensive pain management program that includes recognition, assessment, treatment, and monitoring recommendations.

Summary

An accurate assessment of pain provides the foundation for a successful treatment plan in the older adult. This assessment is often complex, multidimensional, and varies depending on the practice setting where the patient is encountered. Reliance on self-report remains the most reliable measure of the painful complaint. Self-report should be supplemented with existing medical records, information from family members and care givers when possible, and the use of additional instruments available to measure pain-related constructs.

The sheer range and choice of pain-related measurement instruments can be daunting for the clinician. In many cases, particularly when evaluating an elder adult with a chronic pain complaint, the process can be time consuming. Many assessment instruments can be given to the patient before the evaluation process and reviewed with the patient during the examination. One suggestion toward a rational approach to assessment is described previously and includes self-report, the Brief Pain Inventory and the Short Form McGill Pain Questionnaire. Other assessment instruments can be added depending on particular needs of specific populations common to a practice setting. The objective is to make sure the assessment is comprehensive and includes an evaluation of the multidimensional facets of pain in older adults.

The initial evaluation is only the beginning of the assessment process. Ongoing clinical monitoring of treatment outcomes or the development of new clinical findings includes reassessment at appropriate intervals, documentation, and communication of findings to all members of the health team involved in care. By implementing a systematic process in pain assessment clinicians can develop goals and treatment protocols that ultimately optimize pain management in older adults.

References

[1] Hadjistavropoulos T, Herr K, Turk DC, et al. An interdisciplinary expert consensus statement on assessment of pain in older persons. Clin J Pain 2007;23(Suppl 1):S1–43.

[2] Proctor WR, Hirdes JP. Pain and cognitive status among nursing home residents in Canada. Pain Res Manag 2001;6(3):119–25.

[3] Bernabei R, Gambassi G, Lapane K, et al. Management of pain in elderly patients with cancer. SAGE Study Group. Systematic assessment of geriatric drug use via epidemiology. JAMA 1998;279(23):1877–82.

[4] Helme R, Gibson SJ, et al. Pain in older people. In: Crombie I, Croft P, Linton S, editors. Epidemiology of pain. Seattle (WA): IASP Press; 1999. p. 103–12.

[5] Blyth FM, March LM, Brnabic AJ, et al. Chronic pain in Australia: a prevalence study. Pain 2001;89(2–3):127–34.

[6] Martin R, Williams J, Hadjistavropoulos T, et al. A qualitative investigation of seniors' and caregivers' views on pain assessment and management. Can J Nurs Res 2005;37(2):142–64.

[7] Sengstaken EA, King SA. The problems of pain and its detection among geriatric nursing home residents. J Am Geriatr Soc 1993;41(5):541–4.

[8] Helme RD, Gibson SJ. The epidemiology of pain in elderly people. Clin Geriatr Med 2001; 17(3):417–31.

[9] Leveille SG. Musculoskeletal aging. Curr Opin Rheumatol 2004;16(2):114–8.

[10] Weiner DK, Haggerty CL, Kritchevsky SB, et al. How does low back pain impact physical function in independent, well-functioning older adults? Evidence from the health ABC Cohort and implications for the future. Pain Med 2003;4(4):311–20.

[11] Weiner DK, Sakamoto S, Perera S, et al. Chronic low back pain in older adults: prevalence, reliability, and validity of physical examination findings. J Am Geriatr Soc 2006;54(1): 11–20.

[12] McCarberg BH. Rheumatic diseases in the elderly: dealing with rheumatic pain in extended care facilities. Rheum Dis Clin North Am 2007;33(1):87–108.

[13] Bosley BN, Weiner DK, Rudy TE, et al. Is chronic nonmalignant pain associated with decreased appetite in older adults? Preliminary evidence. J Am Geriatr Soc 2004;52(2):247–51.

[14] Magni G, Marchetti M, Moreschi C, et al. Chronic musculoskeletal pain and depressive symptoms in the National Health and Nutrition Examination. I. Epidemiologic follow-up study. Pain 1993;53(2):163–8.

[15] Gallagher RM, Verma S, Mossey J. Chronic pain: sources of late-life pain and risk factors for disability. Geriatrics 2000;55(9):40–7.

[16] Dworkin RH, Turk DC, Farrar JT, et al. Core outcome measures for chronic pain clinical trials: IMMPACT recommendations. Pain 2005;113(1–2):9–19.

[17] Turk DC, Dworkin RH, Allen RR, et al. Core outcome domains for chronic pain clinical trials: IMMPACT recommendations. Pain 2003;106(3):337–45.

[18] Turk DC, Dworkin RH, Burke LB, et al. Developing patient-reported outcome measures for pain clinical trials: IMMPACT recommendations. Pain 2006;125(3):208–15.

[19] AGS Panel on Persistent Pain in Older Persons. The management of persistent pain in older persons [American Geriatrics Society]. J Am Geriatr Soc 2002;50:S205–24.

[20] Feldt KS, Ryden MB, Miles S. Treatment of pain in cognitively impaired compared with cognitively intact older patients with hip-fracture. J Am Geriatr Soc 1998;46(9):1079–85.

[21] Closs SJ, Briggs M. Patients' verbal descriptions of pain and discomfort following orthopaedic surgery. Int J Nurs Stud 2002;39(5):563–72.

[22] Weiner D, Peterson B, Keefe F. Evaluating persistent pain in long term care residents: what role for pain maps? Pain 1998;76(1–2):249–57.

[23] Wynne CF, Ling SM, Remsburg R. Comparison of pain assessment instruments in cognitively intact and cognitively impaired nursing home residents. Geriatr Nurs 2000;21(1): 20–3.

[24] Shanker V. Neurological complications of systemic disease: GI and endrocrine. In: Sirven J, Malamut B, editors. Clinical neurology of the older adult. Philadelphia: Lippincott Williams & Wilkins; 2002. p. 395–404.

[25] Pickholtz J, Malamut B. Cognitive changes associated with normal aging. In: Sirven J, Malamut B, editors. Clinical neurology of the older adult. Philadelphia: Lippincott Williams and Wilkins; 2002. p. 56–64.

[26] Pickholtz J, Malamut B. Cognitive changes associated with normal aging. Philadelphia: Lippincott Williams and Wilkins; 2002.

[27] Herr K. Pain assessment in the older adult with verbal communication skills. In: Gibson SJ, Weiner DK, editors. Progress in pain research and management: pain in older adults, vol. 35. Seattle (WA): IASP Press; 2005. p. 111–33.

[28] Folstein MF, Folstein SE, McHugh PR. Mini-mental state: a practical method for grading the cognitive state of patients for the clinician. J Psychiatr Res 1975;12(3):189–98.

[29] Herr KA, Mobily PR, Smith C. Depression and the experience of chronic back pain: a study of related variables and age differences. Clin J Pain 1993;9(2):104–14.

[30] Turk DC, Okifuji A, Scharff L. Chronic pain and depression: role of perceived impact and perceived control in different age cohorts. Pain 1995;61(1):93–101.

[31] Parmelee PA, Katz IR, Lawton MP. The relation of pain to depression among institutionalized aged. J Gerontol 1991;46(1):P15–21.

[32] Yesavage J, Brink T, Rose T, et al. Development and validation of a geriatric depression scale: a preliminary report. J Psychiatr Res 1983;17:37–49.

[33] Radloff L. The CES-D Scale: a self-report depression scale for research in the general population. Applied Psychological Measurement 1977;1:385–401.

[34] Radloff L, Teri L. The use of CESD with older adults. Clin Gerontol 1986;5:119–35.

[35] Parmelee PA. Measuring mood and psychological function associated with pain in late life. In: Gibson SJ, Weiner DK, editors. Pain in older persons, progress in pain research and management, vol. 35. Seattle (WA): IASP Press; 2005. p. 175–202.

[36] McWilliams LA, Cox BJ, Enns MW. Mood and anxiety disorders associated with chronic pain: an examination in a nationally representative sample. Pain 2003;106(1–2):127–33.

[37] Von Korff M, Crane P, Lane M, et al. Chronic spinal pain and physical-mental comorbidity in the United States: results from the national comorbidity survey replication. Pain 2005; 113(3):331–9.

[38] Beck AT, Epstein N, Brown G, et al. An inventory for measuring clinical anxiety: psychometric properties. J Consult Clin Psychol 1988;56(6):893–7.

[39] Spielberger C, Gorsuch R, Lushene R. Manual for the state-trait anxiety inventory. Palo Alto (CA): Consulting Psychologists Press; 1970.

[40] Keefe FJ, Caldwell DS, Baucom D, et al. Spouse-assisted coping skills training in the management of osteoarthritic knee pain. Arthritis Care Res 1996;9(4):279–91.

[41] Turner JA, Jensen MP, Romano JM. Do beliefs, coping, and catastrophizing independently predict functioning in patients with chronic pain? Pain 2000;85(1–2):115–25.

[42] Brown GK, Nicassio PM. Development of a questionnaire for the assessment of active and passive coping strategies in chronic pain patients. Pain 1987;31(1):53–64.

[43] Snow-Turek AL, Norris MP, Tan G. Active and passive coping strategies in chronic pain patients. Pain 1996;64(3):455–62.

[44] Covic T, Adamson B, Hough M. The impact of passive coping on rheumatoid arthritis pain. Rheumatology (Oxford) 2000;39(9):1027–30.

[45] Keefe FJ, Williams DA. A comparison of coping strategies in chronic pain patients in different age groups. J Gerontol 1990;45(4):P161–5.

[46] Keefe FJ, Caldwell DS, Martinez S, et al. Analyzing pain in rheumatoid arthritis patients: pain coping strategies in patients who have had knee replacement surgery. Pain 1991;46(2): 153–60.

[47] Ersek M, Turner JA, Kemp CA. Use of the chronic pain coping inventory to assess older adults' pain coping strategies. J Pain 2006;7(11):833–42.

[48] Dunn K, Horgas A. Religious and nonreligious coping in older adults experiencing chronic pain. Pain Manag Nurs 2004;5:19–28.

[49] Keefe FJ, Dunsmore J, Burnett R. Behavioral and cognitive-behavioral approaches to chronic pain: recent advances and future directions. J Consult Clin Psychol 1992;60(4): 528–36.

[50] Bandura A. Self-efficacy mechanism in human agency. American Am Psychol 1987;37: 122–47.

[51] Bandura A. Self-efficacy: the exercise of control. New York: Freeman; 1997.

[52] Barry LC, Guo Z, Kerns RD, et al. Functional self-efficacy and pain-related disability among older veterans with chronic pain in a primary care setting. Pain 2003;104(1–2): 131–7.

[53] Reid MC, Williams CS, Gill TM. The relationship between psychological factors and disabling musculoskeletal pain in community-dwelling older persons. J Am Geriatr Soc 2003; 51(8):1092–8.

[54] Turner JA, Ersek M, Kemp C. Self-efficacy for managing pain is associated with disability, depression, and pain coping among retirement community residents with chronic pain. J Pain 2005;6(7):471–9.

[55] Keefe F, Blumenthal J, Baucom D, et al. Effects of spouse-assisted coping skills training and exercise training in patients with osteoarthritic knee pain: a randomized controlled study. Pain 2004;110:539–49.

[56] Keefe F, Caldwell D, Baucom D, et al. Spouse-assisted coping skills training in the management of osteoarthritic knee pain: long term follow up results. Arthritis Care Res 1999;12: 101–11.

[57] Ersek M, Turner JA, McCurry SM, et al. Efficacy of a self-management group intervention for elderly persons with chronic pain. Clin J Pain 2003;19(3):156–67.

[58] Cleeland CS, Ryan KM. Pain assessment: global use of the brief pain inventory. Ann Acad Med Singapore 1994;23(2):129–38.

[59] Melzack R. The short-form McGill pain questionnaire. Pain 1987;30(2):191–7.

[60] Deen G. Back and neck pain. In: Sirven J, Malamut B, editors. Clinical neurology of the older adult. Philadelphia: Lippincott Williams and Wilkins; 2002. p. 191–9.

[61] Tinetti ME. Performance-oriented assessment of mobility problems in elderly patients. J Am Geriatr Soc 1986;34(2):119–26.

[62] Podsiadlo D, Richardson S. The timed Up & Go: a test of basic functional mobility for frail elderly persons. J Am Geriatr Soc 1991;39(2):142–8.

[63] Dodick D, Capobianco D. Headaches. In: Sirven J, Malamut B, editors. Clinical neurology of the older adult. Philadelphia: Lippincott Williams & Wilkins; 2002. p. 176–90.

[64] Andersen G, Vestergaard K, Ingeman-Nielsen M, et al. Incidence of central post-stroke pain. Pain 1995;61(2):187–93.

[65] Benrud-Larson LM, Wegener ST. Chronic pain in neurorehabilitation populations: prevalence, severity and impact. NeuroRehabilitation 2000;14(3):127–37.

[66] Spiera R, Spiera H. Inflammatory disease in older adults: cranial arteritis. Geriatrics 2004; 59(12):25–9 [quiz: 30].

[67] Ardery G, Herr KA, Titler MG, et al. Assessing and managing acute pain in older adults: a research base to guide practice. Medsurg Nurs 2003;12(1):7–18 [quiz: 19].

[68] Schuler M, Njoo N, Hestermann M, et al. Acute and chronic pain in geriatrics: clinical characteristics of pain and the influence of cognition. Pain Med 2004;5(3):253–62.

[69] Pasaro C, Reed B, McCaffery M. Pain in the elderly. 2nd edition. St. Louis (MO): Mosby; 1999.

[70] Marco CA, Plewa MC, Buderer N, et al. Self-reported pain scores in the emergency department: lack of association with vital signs. Acad Emerg Med 2006;13(9):974–9.

[71] Clark L, Jones K, Pennington K. Pain assessment practices with nursing home residents. West J Nurs Res 2004;26(7):733–50.

[72] Kamel HK, Phlavan M, Malekgoudarzi B, et al. Utilizing pain assessment scales increases the frequency of diagnosing pain among elderly nursing home residents. J Pain Symptom Manage 2001;21(6):450–5.

[73] Kaasalainen S, Coker E, Dolovich L, et al. Pain management decision making among long-term care physicians and nurses. West J Nurs Res 2007;29(5):561–80.

[74] American Medical Directors Association (AMDA). Chronic pain management in the long term care setting. Columbia (MD): American Medical Directors Association (AMDA); 2003.

[75] Roland M, Morris R. A study of the natural history of back pain. Part I: development of a reliable and sensitive measure of disability in low-back pain. Spine 1983;8(2): 141–4.

[76] Melzack R. The McGill Pain Questionnaire: major properties and scoring methods. Pain 1975;1:277–99.

[77] Bergh I, Sjostrom B, Oden A, et al. An application of pain rating scales in geriatric patients. Aging Clin Exp Res 2000;12:380–7.

[78] Herr K, Mobily PR. Comparison of selected pain assessment tools for use with the elderly. Appl Nurs Res 1993;6:39–46.

[79] Bieri D, Reeve R, Champion G, et al. The Faces Pain Scale for the self-assessment of the severity of pain experienced by children: initial validation and preliminary investigation for ratio scale properties. Pain 1990;41:139–50.

[80] Wong D, Baker C. Pain in children: comparison of assessment scales. Pediatr Nurs 1988;14: 9–17.

[81] Tait RC, Chibnall JT, Krause S. The Pain Disability Index: psychometric properties. Pain 1990;40:171–82.

[82] Ferrell BA, Stein WM, Beck JC. The Geriatric Pain Measure: validity, reliability and factor analysis. J Am Geriatr Soc 2000;48(12):1669–73.

[83] Kerns RD, Turk DC, Rudy T. The West Haven-Yale Multidimensional Pain Inventory (WHYMPI). Pain 1985;23:345–56.

[84] Gloth F, Scheve A, Stober C, et al. The Functional Pain Scale: reliability, validity and responsiveness in an elderly population. J Am Med Dir Assoc 2001;2:110–4.

[85] Jette A. The Functional Status Index: reliability and validity of a self-report functional disability measure. J Rheumatol Suppl 1987;14(Suppl 15):15–21.

[86] Washburn RA, Smith KW, Jette AM, et al. The Physical Activity Scale for the Elderly (PASE): development and evaluation. J Clin Epidemiol 1993;46(2):153–62.

[87] Fairback JC, Couper J, Davies JB, et al. The Oswestry Back Pain Disability Scale. Physiotherapy 1980;66:271–3.

[88] McConnell S, Kolopack P, Davis AM. The Western Ontario and McMaster Universities Osteoarthritis Index (WOMAC): a review of its utility and measurement properties. Arthritis Rheum 2001;45(5):453–61.

[89] Wheeler AH, Goolkasian P, Baird AC, et al. Development of the Neck Pain and Disability Scale. Item analysis, face, and criterion-related validity. Spine 1999;24(13):1290–4.

[90] Lefebvre M. Cognitive distortion and cognitive errors in depressed psychiatric and low back pain patients. J Consult Clin Psychol 1981;49:517–25.

[91] Gil K, Williams D, Keefe F, et al. The relationship of negative thoughts to pain and psychological distress. Behav Ther 1990;21:349–62.

[92] Yong HH, Gibson SJ, Horne DJ, et al. Development of a pain attitudes questionnaire to assess stoicism and cautiousness for possible age differences. J Gerontol B Psychol Sci Soc Sci 2001;56(5):P279–84.

[93] Sullivan M, Bishop S, Pivik J. The Pain Catastrophizing Scale: development and validation. Psychol Assess 1995;7:524–32.

[94] Nicassio PM, Wallston KA, Callahan LF, et al. The measurement of helplessness in rheumatoid arthritis: the development of the arthritis helplessness index. J Rheumatol 1985; 12(3):462–7.

[95] Lorig K, Chastain RL, Ung E, et al. Development and evaluation of a scale to measure perceived self-efficacy in people with arthritis. Arthritis Rheum 1989;32(1):37–44.

[96] McCracken LM, Zayfert C, Gross RT. The Pain Anxiety Symptoms Scale: development and validation of a scale to measure fear of pain. Pain 1992;50(1):67–73.

[97] Kori S, Miller R, Todd D. Kinesiophobia: a new view of chronic pain behavior. Pain Management 1990;3:35–43.

[98] Cook AJ, Brawer PA, Vowles KE. The fear-avoidance model of chronic pain: validation and age analysis using structural equation modeling. Pain 2006;121(3):195–206.

[99] Burwinkle T, Robinson JP, Turk DC. Fear of movement: factor structure of the Tampa scale of kinesiophobia in patients with fibromyalgia syndrome. J Pain 2005;6(6):384–91.

[100] Lachman ME, Howland J, Tennstedt S, et al. Fear of falling and activity restriction: the survey of activities and fear of falling in the elderly (SAFE). J Gerontol B Psychol Sci Soc Sci 1998;53(1):P43–50.

[101] Rosenstiel AK, Keefe FJ. The use of coping strategies in chronic low back pain patients: relationship to patient characteristics and current adjustment. Pain 1983;17(1):33–44.

[102] Jensen MP, Turner JA, Romano JM, et al. The Chronic Pain Coping Inventory: development and preliminary validation. Pain 1995;60(2):203–16.

[103] Felton BJ, Revenson TA. Coping with chronic illness: a study of illness controllability and the influence of coping strategies on psychological adjustment. J Consult Clin Psychol 1984; 52(3):343–53.

[104] Felton BJ, Revenson TA, Hinrichsen GA. Stress and coping in the explanation of psychological adjustment among chronically ill adults. Soc Sci Med 1984;18(10):889–98.

[105] Folkman S, Lazarus RS. If it changes it must be a process: study of emotion and coping during three stages of a college examination. J Pers Soc Psychol 1985;48(1):150–70.

ELSEVIER
SAUNDERS

CLINICS IN
GERIATRIC
MEDICINE

Clin Geriatr Med 24 (2008) 237–262

Assessment of Pain in the Nonverbal or Cognitively Impaired Older Adult

Karen Bjoro, PhD(c), RN[a,b,*],
Keela Herr, PhD, RN, FAAN, AGSF[a]

[a]College of Nursing, The University of Iowa, 101 Nursing Building, Iowa City, IA 52242, USA
[b]Department of Research, Nursing Unit, Ulleval University Hospital, Kirkeveien 166,
0407 Oslo, Norway

Pain is a highly subjective and personal experience. Self-report is widely accepted as the most reliable source of information on an individual's pain experience and is considered to be the gold standard in most populations [1,2]. Yet, older adults with severe cognitive impairment or who are unconscious or intubated during an episode of severe critical illness are unable to communicate their pain experience. Inability to use verbal language represents a major barrier to pain assessment and treatment. For these individuals alternative approaches to pain assessment involving observation of pain behaviors and proxy pain report are necessary.

The ability to use language is a comprehensive and complex behavior acquired in early childhood. Primary faculties of language include speaking, signing, and language comprehension, whereas reading and writing are secondary abilities [3]. With language impairment (eg, aphasia, dysphasia) ability to communicate orally, through signs, or in writing, or the ability to understand such communications may be severely compromised. Language impairment (eg, aphasia, dysphasia) is associated with many medical illnesses and clinical states, as listed below. Loss of ability to communicate is a core feature of many types of cognitive impairment (eg, dementia and delirium), and occurs frequently with severe critical illness and at end of life with the naturally occurring deterioration in cognition resulting from ensuing death or sedation.

---

* Corresponding author. Department of Research, Nursing Unit, Ulleval University Hospital, Kirkeveien 166, 0407 Oslo, Norway.
    E-mail address: karen.bjoro@ulleval.no (K. Bjoro).

Dementias
Delirium
Cerebrovascular accident
State of unconsciousness, advanced life support, intubation
Severe depression
Psychosis
Mental disability
Coma, persistent vegetative state
Encephalopathy
Terminal illness

This article reviews the current basis for pain assessment in three nonverbal populations: (1) those with advanced dementia, (2) those with delirium, and (3) those experiencing an episode of critical illness unable to communicate because of unconscious state or presence of an endotracheal tube. General principles of pain assessment and specific recommendations for pain assessment of nonverbal older adults are discussed. Finally, a selection of behavioral pain assessment tools for use with these nonverbal older adults is critiqued.

Challenge of dementia for pain assessment

Dementia is one of the most frequent causes of cognitive impairment in older adults with a forecast worldwide increase in incidence from 25 million in 2000 to 114 million by 2050 [4]. Dementia involves the development of multiple cognitive deficits manifested by impaired memory and involving cognitive disturbances, loss of language, ability to recognize or identify objects, and executive function [5]. As dementia progresses to advanced stages individuals become increasingly dependent in all activities of daily living, often requiring skilled nursing care.

The burden of dementia in the older adult population is compounded by a considerable pain burden [6]. In institutionalized older adults with dementia, pain or potentially painful conditions are common, with prevalence estimates ranging between 49% and 83% [7,8]. One large-scale nursing home study documented that one half of the residents reported having pain in the past week and a fourth experienced pain daily [9]. Moreover, similar prevalence of pain was documented in subgroups of cognitively intact and impaired residents. The most common pain-associated conditions in the cognitively impaired residents were arthritis; previous hip fracture; osteoporosis; pressure ulcers; depression; and history of a recent fall, unsteady gait, and verbally abusive behavior [9].

The severity of cognitive impairment and progression of language deficit vary by type and stage of disease, environmental factors, and individual characteristics. In Alzheimer's disease (AD), which accounts for over half of dementia cases, memory deficit is the presenting symptom with language impairments developing gradually over the course of the illness [10]. Typically, AD patients are fluent until the middle to late stages of the disease, whereas global language disturbance and mutism are generally present in the end stage of AD. With vascular dementia, the second most prevalent type of dementia, the trajectory of language impairment resembles that observed in AD [11]. By comparison, individuals with frontotemporal dementia (behavioral type) and primary progressive aphasia show earlier onset of language impairment and more rapid decline [10]. Subtype of dementia also seems to impact pain response. In frontotemporal dementia a decrease in affective pain response has been documented, which could be explained by atrophy of the prefrontal cortex; by contrast, with vascular dementia an increase in affective response is reported that may be related to white matter lesions and deafferentiation in these patients [12].

Neuropathologic processes in dementia seriously impact the ability of those with advanced stages of disease to communicate pain. Only a few studies have investigated the relationship between dementia and the neuropathology of pain, however, and these are limited to experimental pain studies in individuals with AD. Whereas sensory discriminatory aspects of pain are processed in the lateral pain system (eg, lateral thalamus), motivational affective aspects are processed in the medial pain system (eg, anterior cingulate gyrus, hippocampus) [13,14]. Noxious stimuli transmitted by the lateral pain system are interpreted in the somatosensory cortex, involving areas of the brain that are relatively unaffected by AD neuropathology. This explains the finding that sensory aspects of pain remain intact in individuals with AD. Nevertheless, the lateral pain system does show some functional decline as evidenced by elevated pain threshold and report of less intense pain in those with AD. By contrast, the medial pain system is severely affected by pathologic processes in AD [12,15]. Affective pain response (eg, pain tolerance) was significantly increased in individuals with AD compared with those without dementia [12]. Empiric studies indicate that older adults with dementia are not less sensitive to pain, but that they may fail to interpret sensations as painful.

Despite these findings, evidence suggests that older adults with advanced dementia underreport pain relative to those who are cognitively intact. Research studies have documented a decrease in the number of pain complaints with increasing severity of cognitive impairment in older adults with dementia [16,17]. Inability to communicate is a major barrier to adequate pain assessment and treatment in older adults with advanced dementia. Cognitively impaired older adults hospitalized with hip fracture received significantly less opioid analgesia than those with less or no impairment [18,19]. In the nursing home setting pain is documented less frequently in residents unable to communicate their pain even though they have a similar number of painful diagnoses [9,20,21]. Moreover, less analgesia is prescribed and administered for cognitively impaired nursing home residents, even when the impaired residents have similar numbers of painful diagnoses as cognitively intact residents [22,23]. Inability to communicate in older adults with dementia is a major barrier to both assessment and treatment. Language impairment is also common in delirium.

Challenge of delirium for pain assessment

Delirium is a form of transient cognitive impairment often accompanied by loss of ability to communicate effectively. The incidence of delirium in older adults ranges from 16% to 62% with hip fracture [24], 62% in the ICU [25], 25% to 45% in older cancer patients [26], and approximately 22% in nursing home residents [27].

Delirium is characterized by recent onset of fluctuating awareness and inability to focus attention, change in cognition (eg, memory deficit, disorientation), or perceptual disturbance, and the presence of an underlying organic illness [5]. There are three clinical subtypes of delirium: (1) hyperactive, (2) hypoactive, and (3) mixed [28]. Language disturbance in delirium is characteristically manifested by impaired ability to articulate, name objects, write, or even speak. Speech may be rambling and irrelevant, or pressured and incoherent, with unpredictable shifting from subject to subject [5]. Although older adults with delirium may be able to speak, the content may be incomprehensible.

Although the pathophysiology of delirium remains unclear, there is general agreement that delirium etiology is multifactorial [29,30]. Inouye and Charpentier [29] proposed that delirium may develop in a vulnerable individual because of the interaction of predisposing and precipitating risk factors. Predisposing factors (eg, high age, dementia, and multiple chronic diseases) increase the vulnerability of an individual to noxious factors that interact with underlying predisposing factors to precipitate the onset of delirium. Whereas many potential precipitating factors have been identified (eg, dehydration, electrolyte disturbance, polypharmacy, infection, hypoxia), delirium onset has also been linked to antecedent pain in hip fracture patients [31], medical patients [32], and older adults undergoing elective surgery [33,34]. Many of the analgesics (eg, meperidine [31,35]) and other adjuvant medications used to treat pain (eg, benzodiazepine [35]), however, can also trigger onset of delirium. The relationship between pain, pain treatment, and delirium is complex and unclear.

Pain assessment in older adults with delirium is extremely challenging. No diagnostic tests exist to determine the presence of either pain or delirium. Identification of pain in nonverbal older adults and delirium both rely on observation of behavioral presentation. Moreover, there is considerable overlap between delirium behaviors and nonverbal pain behaviors. Liptzin and Levkoff [36] used behavioral items on the Delirium Symptom Interview [37] to observe hypoactive and hyperactive behaviors of patients with delirium (Table 1). Interestingly, many behavioral symptoms of delirium also occur on a comprehensive list of nonverbal pain behaviors (Table 2) (eg, wandering, verbally abusive behavior, resistiveness to care).

Table 1
Delirium subtype and associated potential behavioral symptoms

Delirium subtype	Behavioral symptoms
Hyperactive	Hypervigilance
	Restlessness
	Fast or loud speech
	Irritability
	Combativeness
	Impatience
	Swearing
	Singing
	Laughing
	Uncooperative
	Euphoric
	Anger
	Wandering
	Easy startling
	Fast motor responses
	Distractability
	Tangentiality
	Nightmares
	Persistent thoughts
Hypoactive	Unawareness
	Decreased alertness
	Sparse or slow speech
	Lethargic
	Slowed movements
	Staring
	Apathy

Data from Liptzin B, Levkoff SE. An empirical study of delirium subtypes. Br J Psychiatry 1992;161:843–845.

Few studies have investigated pain assessment in older adults with ongoing delirium. One study showed that physicians and nurses were likely to misinterpret agitation as an expression of pain in patients with agitated delirium in whom the pain was well controlled before and after the delirium episode [38]. Further, it is unclear whether available behavioral pain tools may assist in pain detection in older adults during episodes of delirium. Only one pain assessment tool has been developed for use with this particular patient population; however, initial testing of the tool was conducted in cognitively intact older adults undergoing orthopedic surgery, and not in those with cognitive impairments [39].

The relationships between pain and delirium are complex and unclear. Although improved pain treatment may reduce the occurrence of delirium in older adults, there is a gap in the literature regarding assessment of pain in patients with delirium. It may not be possible to identify pain definitively by behavioral presentation in patients with delirium and may require alternative approaches to pain assessment, such as analgesic trial, addressed in later sections of this article.

Table 2
Common pain behaviors in cognitively impaired older persons

Behavior	Examples
Facial expressions	Slight frown, sad, frightened face
	Grimacing, wrinkled forehead, closed or tightened eyes
	Any distorted expression
	Rapid blinking
Verbalizations, vocalizations	Sighing, moaning, groaning
	Grunting, chanting, calling out
	Noisy breathing
	Asking for help
	Verbal abusiveness
Body movements	Rigid, tense body posture, guarding
	Fidgeting
	Increased pacing, rocking
	Restricted movement
	Gait or mobility changes
Changes in interpersonal interactions	Aggressive, combative, resists care
	Decreased social interactions
	Socially inappropriate, disruptive
	Withdrawn
Changes in activity patterns or routines	Refusing food, appetite change
	Increase in rest periods
	Sleep, rest pattern changes
	Sudden cessation of common routines
	Increased wandering
Mental status changes	Crying or tears
	Increased confusion
	Irritability or distress

From American Geriatrics Society Panel on Persistent Pain in Older Adults. The management of persistent pain in older persons. J Am Geriatr Soc 2002;50:S211; with permission.

Challenge of severe critical illness for pain assessment

Older adults have increased prevalence of comorbid illness and trauma and account for more than 60% of all ICU days [40]. During episodes of severe critical illness older people may lose the ability to speak because of unconscious state, presence of an endotracheal tube, or fatigue.

Many older adults die in the ICU [41]. Patients able to report the ICU experience in retrospect have indicated that endotracheal intubation, mechanical ventilation, and consequent inability to speak are extremely stressful events [41–43]. Pain and inability to speak were reported to be moderately to extremely bothersome. Endotracheal suctioning is a particularly painful procedure, and the stressful experience associated with the endotracheal tube was strongly associated with subjects' experiencing spells of terror [42].

Sources of pain during episodes of critical illness include existing medical condition; traumatic injuries; surgical or medical procedure; invasive instrumentation; blood draws; and other routine care, such as turning, positioning, drain and catheter removal, and wound care [44–46]. Adult patients have described the experience of pain in critical illness as a constant baseline aching pain with intermittent procedure-related pain that is experienced as sharp, stinging, stabbing, shooting, and awful pain [45]. Although most studies have been conducted with younger patients, it should be assumed that nonverbal older adults also experience these sensations.

Identification of pain in nonverbal older patients who are unable to communicate their pain and discomfort because of critical illness requires astute observational skill. Moreover, the complexity of detecting pain is confounded by the overhanging threat of delirium that occurs in approximately 62% of older adults in the ICU [25].

The inability of nonverbal populations to communicate pain and discomfort represents a major barrier to adequate pain assessment and treatment. The evidence indicates the urgent need to improve methods of detecting and managing pain in these vulnerable populations and is addressed in the following section.

Approaches to pain assessment in nonverbal older adults

Assessment of pain is a critical component of a comprehensive approach to pain management in all populations. The purpose of pain assessment is to detect the presence and source of pain, identify any comorbidities requiring attention, determine the effect of pain on function, and collect data on which to base individual treatment plans [6]. Achievement of these goals is challenging in nonverbal older adults. Nevertheless, general principles can guide approaches to pain identification, measurement, and continuous monitoring and selection of specific pain assessment strategies in nonverbal older adults.

The American Society for Pain Management Nursing recently published recommendations for pain assessment in nonverbal individuals [47]. This comprehensive, hierarchical strategy includes five key principles to guide pain assessment in nonverbal populations: (1) obtain self-report if at all possible, (2) investigate for possible pathologies that could produce pain, (3) observe for behaviors that may indicate pain, (4) solicit surrogate report, and (5) use analgesics to evaluate whether pain management causes a reduction in the behavioral indicators thought to be related to pain [47]. These principles reflect a decision-making process illustrated in Fig. 1 that may guide and support health care clinicians and are discussed in greater depth in the following section.

Obtain self-report

Attempts should be made to obtain self-report of pain from all patients. The ability of cognitively impaired patients to report their pain consistently

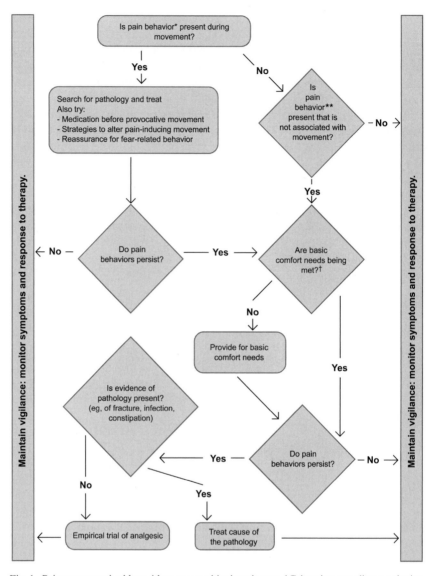

Fig. 1. Pain assessment in elders with severe cognitive impairment. *Grimacing, guarding, combative-ness, groaning with movement, resisting care. **Agitation, fidgeting, sleep disturbance, diminished ap-petite, irritability, reclusiveness, disruptive behavior, rigidity, rapid blinking. †Toileting, thirst, hunger, visual or hearing impairment. (*Adapted from* Reuben DB, Herr KA, Pacala JT, et al. Geriatrics at your fingertips: 2007-2008 edition. New York: The American Geriatrics Society; 2007; with permission.)

and accurately varies widely across levels of cognitive impairment [48]. Research indicates that individuals with mild and moderate dementia and even some with severe dementia are able to self-report [7,48–50]. Even a lim-ited yes or no response to a query regarding pain presence is important information regarding the patient's own pain experience.

With increasing cognitive impairment, ability reliably to use self-report instruments wanes. Although no clear method has been identified to address reliability in using self-report instruments, Buffum and colleagues [51] described a Pain Screening Tool, an approach developed for evaluating cognitive ability reliably to complete pain intensity scales. Patients are asked to provide a number from 0 to 3 and a word to describe their pain. Following 1 minute of distracting conversation, the respondent is asked to recall the number and word. Patients receive one point each for being able to provide an initial number and word and one half point each for recalling the number and the word. Only respondents who score a three are identified as providing reliable pain reports.

Strategies that increase the likelihood of obtaining a self-report of pain from a cognitively impaired individual may include use of a modified verbal rating scale with limited number of descriptors, careful instruction on tool use and repetition, focus on the individual's current pain rather than past pain experience, and adaptation of tools to compensate for possible sensory impairments [48,52]. Despite these efforts, however, many patients' impairments are severe enough to require alternative approaches to assessment.

Search for potential causes of pain

Pathologic conditions should be considered as a potential cause of pain and discomfort in the assessment process. History and general physical evaluation, examination of any painful regions, and consideration of any pain medication regimen provide essential information for clinical decisions. Musculoskeletal and neurologic conditions are among the most common causes of pain in older adults and should be given priority in the clinical examination. Moreover, evaluation of the patient's cognitive status is a crucial element of geriatric-focused pain assessment because both acute and chronic pain can impact cognition. When pain-associated pathologies are identified, presence of pain may be assumed and appropriate pain intervention strategies should be implemented. Pain should be treated preemptively before initiation of any procedures known to cause pain [1,47]. A change in behavior should initiate a search for any acute problems as a source of pain or discomfort (eg, pneumonia, urinary tract infection, or a recent fall). Detailed guidelines with recommendations for assessment of pain pathology in older adults are available [6].

Observe for behaviors that may indicate pain

When older adults are unable to communicate presence of pain because of cognitive impairments, unconsciousness, or severe critical illness, reliance on external signs of pain, such as nonverbal behaviors and physiologic changes, becomes a necessary approach to pain detection. The American Geriatrics Society Panel on Persistent Pain in Older Adults [2] has compiled a comprehensive list of nonverbal behaviors observed in older adults with cognitive impairment with six categories of pain behavioral indicators: (1)

facial expressions, (2) verbalizations and vocalizations, (3) body movements, (4) changes in interpersonal interactions, (5) changes in activity patterns or routines, and (6) mental status change (see Table 2). This framework provides a valuable resource for evaluating the relevance and comprehensiveness of behaviors included on a particular behavioral pain tool for use with older adults [53].

Observational approaches to pain assessment rely on interpretation of behaviors. The inherent subjectivity involved in observational approaches represents challenges to the reliability and validity of pain assessments. Important issues for consideration when using behavioral observation to detect pain or when selecting a behavioral pain tool are summarized in Table 3. The following provides recommendations that may maximize observational pain assessment approaches in nonverbal older adults.

Behavioral indicators for pain assessment must be appropriate to the patient population, setting, and type of pain problems encountered. The shorter behavioral pain tools tend to be direct observation focused including specific behaviors that may be observed in a direct encounter by trained observers (eg, grimacing, guarding, restlessness, moaning, fighting the ventilator) [54,55]. The patient may be observed for a specified period and activity for the presence or absence, intensity, or frequency of pain behaviors [54,56]. Shorter behavioral tools require no previous history with the patient, an advantage in the acute-care setting. Longer pain scales are more comprehensive including more subtle behavioral indicators in addition to those commonly observed. Such items as changes in activity patterns or routines, interpersonal interactions, or mental status require involvement of family and caregivers familiar with the patient's baseline or typical behaviors. Longer tools may be more appropriate in long-term care settings where patients may be observed over time while performing everyday activities.

With chronic pain states, changes in physiologic indicators are often not observed. In acute pain situations physiologic and behavioral indicators may increase temporarily, but these changes may be attributed to underlying physiologic conditions and medications. Changes in vital signs are not reliable as single indicators of pain, but changes in physiologic indicators (eg, blood pressure, pulse, oxygen saturation) should be considered a cue to begin further assessment for pain or other stressors. Moreover, absence of increased vital signs does not indicate absence of pain [57,58].

Conditions of behavioral observation are also important to ensure reliability of assessments. Observation of behaviors should occur during movement or activity that is likely to elicit a pain response if pain is present. Studies have demonstrated that observation of pain behaviors at rest is misleading and can result in false judgments that pain is absent leading to underdetection and undertreatment [18,54,59,60]. Moreover, serial observations should be performed under similar circumstances (eg, time of day and activity performed) to ensure comparability of behavioral pain assessments over time.

Table 3
Key issues in behavioral pain assessment in older adults with cognitive impairment

Issue	Key considerations
Specific versus Subtle behaviors	Specific behaviors are obvious and commonly observed in pain states (eg, facial expressions, verbalizations or vocalizations, body movements) [2].
	Subtle behaviors reflect change from usual individual behavioral pattern and are less obvious pain indicators (eg, changes in interpersonal interactions, activity patterns, or mental status) [2].
	Subtle behaviors require interpretation and validation that pain is the etiology.
Direct observation versus Surrogate report	Specific, obvious indicators may be observed directly. No prior history with the patient is required.
	Subtle behaviors of change from baseline require reassessment over time by individuals familiar with the patient.
	Use of surrogate reporting requires caution because of evidence of disagreements between self-report of pain by cognitively impaired individuals and proxy report [84–87].
Pain presence versus Severity	Patient self-report and proxy report of pain severity show increasing disagreement with increasing severity of cognitive impairment [50].
	Evidence documents surrogate or proxy ability to recognize pain presence but not intensity [84].
	Professional caregivers tend to underestimate patient pain severity [84,86,88].
	Family members tend to overestimate patient pain severity and level of discomfort [89].
	A behavioral pain tool score is not the same as a pain intensity rating. Pain behavior tool score and score on pain intensity ratings should not be compared [90].
Sensitivity versus Specificity	A comprehensive indicator set including obvious and less obvious pain behaviors increases sensitivity of behavioral tools to detect pain when present [91].
	A narrow indicator set with only obvious indicators increases specificity of behavioral tools to rule out pain when pain is not present, but are less sensitive in detecting pain in those with less obvious pain presentation [91].
Screening versus Diagnostic certainty	Behavioral pain assessment may assist in screening for presence of pain, but does not provide diagnostic certainty regarding exact nature and cause of possible pain to guide treatment [64–66,68].
	In situations in which uncertainty prevails, an empiric analgesic trial is warranted as a pain assessment strategy [1,6,47].

Solicit support of surrogate reporters

In the absence of pain self-report, surrogate observation is an important source of information. Family members or others who know the patient well (eg, spouse, child, caregiver) should be encouraged to provide information regarding usual and past behaviors and assist in identification of subtle, less obvious changes in behavior that may indicate pain presence. In long-term care the certified nursing assistant is a key health care provider who has been shown to be effective in recognizing the presence of pain [61,62]. In settings in which health care providers do not have a history with the patient, family members are likely to be the caregivers with the most familiarity with typical pain behaviors or changes in usual activities that might suggest pain presence. A family member's report of their impression of a patient's pain and response to an intervention should be included as one component of pain assessment that includes multiple sources of information. When engaging multiple care providers and surrogates in pain screening procedures, training is important to safeguard reliability of behavioral observations. Moreover, when introducing new behavioral tools to the clinical setting, interrater reliability between caregivers should be established initially and on a regular basis to calibrate observations, reducing subjectivity and potential for bias associated with this method.

Conduct an analgesic trial

If after following the initial steps in this multifaceted approach to pain assessment behaviors that may indicate pain persist, an analgesic trial is warranted. The underlying supposition is that any reduction in behaviors following analgesic intervention is related to improved pain control. Early unblinded trials provided preliminary support for this approach [63]. Buffum and colleagues [64] did not demonstrate significant changes in agitated behavior thought to be pain-related in persons with advanced dementia; however, the acetaminophen dose was only 2600 mg/day. In a randomized controlled trial evaluating low-dose opioids in persons with dementia, Manfredi and colleagues [65] reported decreased agitation in the over-85 age group and suggested that less response in the younger old group could be related to low dosing of analgesic. In a recent double-blind crossover randomized controlled trial with patients with dementia receiving 3000 mg/day of acetaminophen, Chibnall and colleagues [66] demonstrated increased levels of social activity and interaction compared with times receiving placebo. An analgesic trial is an integrated component of the Serial Trial Intervention, a clinical protocol developed by Kovach and colleagues [67] that uses a systematic method for assessing and treating potential pain related behaviors in patients with severe dementia. A recent randomized controlled trial of the Serial Trial Intervention demonstrated significantly less discomfort and behavioral symptoms returning to baseline more frequently in the treatment group and has been shown to be effective in increasing recognition and treatment of pain in persons with dementia [68]. Although analgesic trial is a promising approach, selecting and titrating analgesics for this purpose has not been clearly explicated or studied. The use of an analgesic trial as a means to evaluate pain as the cause of potential pain-related behaviors requires further investigation, but is likely an important step in the process of recognizing and validating pain in those presenting with atypical pain behaviors.

Summary

This section has outlined key components of a comprehensive approach to pain assessment in nonverbal older adults. A multifaceted approach is recommended that combines direct observation of behaviors, family and caregiver input, and evaluation of response to treatment. A standardized behavioral pain tool may be used as one component of a comprehensive approach to pain assessment and is addressed in the following section.

Behavioral pain assessment tools for use with older adults

During the past 10 years, a number of standardized tools for pain assessment based on observation of behaviors have been developed for use with nonverbal older adult populations. Several reviews of available tools [53,69–72] have indicated that although there are tools with potential, there is currently no tool that has sufficiently strong reliability and validity to support recommendation for broad adoption in clinical practice. Moreover, reviews have called for further tool testing in larger samples or in diverse clinical settings. In an earlier comprehensive review, Herr and coworkers [53] critiqued 10 tools for use with nonverbal adults with advanced dementia based on published reports of psychometric data. Since the publication of this review, some tools have undergone further testing and development. In the following discussion a selection of tools is presented with updated critiques. Also included are two recently developed tools for use with critically ill adult patients who are unconscious or intubated that have not previously been critiqued for relevance, reliability, and validity for use with critically ill older adults. Table 4 provides an overview of characteristics of the selected tools with presentation of tool items and scoring range, reliability, and validity and clinical utility.

The Checklist of Nonverbal Pain Indicators (CNPI) [18,54], developed to measure pain in cognitively impaired older adults, includes six conceptually sound behavioral items commonly observed in direct observation situations. Initial tool testing supports reliability and validity for tool use in acute care, although internal consistencies were low suggesting the need for further testing. In tool evaluation in Norwegian nursing homes test-retest and interrater reliabilities reported were low to moderate when administered by various categories of nursing personnel as an element of daily care, and concurrent validity was supported [73]. In another recent study in long-term care, sensitivity of the CNPI was moderate, whereas at the same time nearly half the residents who reported having pain showed no pain behaviors on the CNPI, giving rise to concerns about the ability of the tool to detect pain in those unable to report. Because the CNPI lacks indicators of subtle behaviors, the tool's ability to detect pain in those with less obvious behavioral presentation is questioned. This tool may be more appropriate for use in acute care; however, additional testing in larger and more acute-care samples is needed.

Table 4
Characteristics of selected behavioral pain assessment tools for nonverbal older adults with dementia or severe critical illness (unconscious or intubated)

Tools for nonverbal older adults who have severe critical illness

Tool name	Items/scoring range	Reliability	Validity	Feasibility/utility	Summary
CNPI [18,54,73,91]	6 items: nonverbal vocalizations, facial grimacing or wincing, bracing, rubbing, restlessness, vocal complaints. Items scored present or absent at rest and on movement Total score range 0–12	Internal consistency: 0.54–0.64 Interrater reliability: κ = 0.62–0.82 Percent agreement: 74%–94% κ = 0.45–0.69 Test-retest: 34%–41% κ = 0.23–0.66	Moderate discriminant validity supported by higher scores on movement versus at rest Convergent validity supported by moderate correlations with VDS with movement, but only weak correlation at rest In long-term care: Sensitivity: 55% Specificity: 85% Convergent validity supported by significant positive relationship between self-report of pain intensity and CNPI score. Concurrent validity supported by positive correlation with nurse rated VAS	Language of original: English Translations: Norwegian, Dutch Easy to use Scoring instructions provided Score interpretation unclear Tested in acute care and long-term care.	CNPI includes only common obvious behaviors observed by direct observation. Tool seems to lack ability to detect pain in individuals with less common pain presentation (eg, nursing home residents). CNPI seems more appropriate for pain assessment in acute care and procedural pain situations.

| Doloplus-2 [49,74–76] | 10 items, three dimensions of somatic (N = 5), psychomotor (N = 2), psychosocial (N = 3) Score range: 0–30 Reflects progression of experienced pain, not current pain experience | Internal consistency: Total scale: 0.82 Subscales: Somatic: 0.63–0.7 Psychomotor: 0.7–0.8 Psychosocial: 0.58–0.63 Interrater reliability: Not established Test-retest: Not established | Convergent validity supported by moderate positive correlations with self-report of pain on VAS ($r = .65$) and on VAS, VRS and FPS ($r = .31–.40$). Predictive validity supported by significant prediction of expert rated NRS-11 score. Four items explained 62% of the expert score. Four items explained 68% of the variance of the expert rated pain score. Sensitivity: 71% Specificity: 76% Concurrent validity indicated by moderate correlations with PACSLAC, PAINAD, a nurse-rated VAS, and an expert rated VAS. | Language of original: French Translations: Dutch, Norwegian, English English translation issues are evident and English version is not tested. Estimated time to complete 5 min Tool manual is clear. Tool evaluation by nurses shows the tool is difficult to score and interpret. | Psychosocial subscale seems to need revision based on psychometric results. Nurses report tool is difficult to score and interpret. English tool version needs testing in English speaking population. |

(continued on next page)

Table 4 (continued)

Tools for nonverbal older adults who have severe critical illness

Tool name	Items/scoring range	Reliability	Validity	Feasibility/utility	Summary
PACSLAC [75,77]	60 items, four dimensions: Facial expression (N = 13) Activity/body movements (N = 20) Social/personality/mood (N = 12) Physiologic/eating/sleeping/vocal (N = 15) Score range 0–60	Internal consistency: Retrospecitve data: 0.85 Total tool: 0.62–0.84 Subscales: 0.12–0.76 Interrater reliability: 0.92 Test-retest: Good intrarater reliabilities	Discriminant validity supported by: Moderate ability to differentiate between pain, calm, and distress events based on rater memory Ability to differentiate levels of pain: at rest, during influenza vaccination and during mobilization and bathing Congruent validity supported by significant positive correlations with PAINAD, self-report and proxy rating on VAS	Language of original: English Translations: Dutch Appears easy to use; Estimated time to complete 5 min Nurses report that some items on the tool are redundant	Tool most preferred by nurses when compared with PAINAD and Doloplus 2 Promising tool but item reduction and subscale revisions needed
PACSLAC-D-Revised [92]	24 items, three subscales: Facial and vocal expressions (N = 10) Resistance/defense (N = 6) Social-emotional aspects/mood (N = 8) Score range 0–24	Internal consistency: Total tool: 0.82–0.86 Subscales: 0.72–0.82 Interrater reliability: Not yet established Test-retest: Not yet evaluated	Correlation with original PACSLAC suggests validity is retained	Available in Dutch and English translation Clinical utility not yet evaluated	Promising preliminary tool needs prospective testing in independent sample Testing in English speaking population needed

| PAINAD [75,78–80,93–96] | 5 items: breathing, negative vocalizations, facial expression, body language, consolability Score range 0–10 | Internal consistency: 0.50–0.67 0.69–0.74 Interrater reliability: r = 0.82–0.97 0.75–0.81 Test-retest: r = 0.90 (P < .001) Time interval: morning/evening skift scores r = 0.88 (interval: 15 d) r = 0.89 | Discriminant validity supported by 1) moderate ability to differentiate pleasant and aversive activities 2) before and after pain medication 3) ability to differentiate levels of pain: at rest, during influenza vaccination and during mobilization and bathing Ability to detect change before and after pain medication in treatment group versus controls Moderate effect size Convergent validity indicated by positive correlations with DS-DAT, PACSLAC, and nurse-rated VAS Scores on the DS-DAT decreased following pain intervention Divergent validity indicated by no correlation with MMSE and GDS and Cornell Depression Scale and AMT score | Language of original: English. Translations: Dutch, German, Italian Requires 5-min observation period Uncertainty about when to implement consolability item Nurses evaluate tool as too concise | Actual interval time for test-retest not reported Measurement of pain severity by observation of behaviors not supported in the literature, although tool seems to discriminate between levels of pain Usefulness of breathing and consolability items for pain detection is questioned Concerning validity there was no indication as to whether raters were blind to the intervention, and subjects were not randomly allocated to treatment or control group. |

(continued on next page)

Table 4 (continued)

Tools for nonverbal older adults who have severe critical illness

Tool name	Items/scoring range	Reliability	Validity	Feasibility/utility	Summary
BPS [81–83]	Three behavioral items: facial expression movements of upper limbs compliance with ventilation Score range 3–12	Interrater reliability: 0.64–0.72 Interrater reliability: κ=0.74 (P<.01) Interrater reliability: r²=0.91–0.89 Percent agreement: 36%–91% Test-retest: Not established	Discriminant validity indicated by significantly higher BPS scores during painful procedure (repositioning) compared with rest periods and nonsignificant increase in average BPS during a less painful procedure (eye care) The higher the sedation/analgesia administered, the lower the BPS value and BPS change Factor analysis supports content validity in adults Support for tool ability to detect change in clinical status and detect painful procedures is indicated by large effect size for both subscale scores and for total BPS scores Despite significant increase in physiologic variables (heart rate and mean arterial blood pressure) between rest and painful procedure times, correlations among BPS score and heart rate and blood pressure were not significant. Significant negative correlations with Ramsay sedation scale. The higher the sedation level, the lower the BPS scores	Language of original: French Translations: English Appears easy to use; Requires 4 min on average to complete Reported less difficulty agreeing on pain level when pain level was low, but greater when assessing increased pain level Interpretation of tool score unclear	Psychometric evaluation largely based on observations as unit of analysis rather than patients Internal consistency is variable. Interrater reliability varies widely across studies. Tool not evaluated in sample of older adults

CPOT [55]	4 items: facial expression, body movements, muscle tension, compliance to ventilator if the patient is intubated or vocalization if extubated. Score range 0–8	Internal consistency: Not established. Interrater reliability: $\kappa=0.52$–0.88. Test-retest: Not established	Criterion validity with intubated or conscious patients indicated by significantly higher CPOT scores for patients reporting pain presence compared with lack of pain during positioning, at rest, and recovery postprocedure. Moderate criterion validity in extubated conscious patients indicated by moderate correlations between CPOT scores and self-reported pain intensity scores during positioning, at rest, and recovery postprocedure. Moderate ability to discriminate pain indicated by significantly higher CPOT scores during positioning than during rest in three situations: (1) intubated and unconscious, (2) intubated and conscious, and (3) extubated and conscious	Language of original tool: French. Requires 1 min observation period. Interpretation of score unclear	Evidence of internal consistency is needed. Evaluation of French tool conducted in French-speaking population. Evaluation in English is needed. Tool evaluation in older adult samples is warranted. Tool evaluation in larger samples and with a variety of conditions is needed

Abbreviations: BPS, behavioral pain scale; CNPI, checklist of nonverbal pain indicators; CPOT, critical care pain observation tool; FPS, faces pain scale; PACSLAC, Pain assessment checklist for seniors with limited ability to communicate; PAINAD, Pain in advanced dementia; VAS, visual analog scale; VDS, verbal descriptor scale; VRS, verbal rating scale.

The Doloplus 2 [74] is a French tool developed for multidimensional assessment of pain in nonverbal older adults. Psychometric evaluations are available based on French, Dutch, and Norwegian speaking populations, but not English. The Doloplus 2 addresses many key indicators noted in the literature and American Geriatric Society guidelines. Doloplus reflects progression of experienced pain, not current pain experience; intrarater and interrater reliability of the tool represent a particular challenge and have not yet been adequately established. Although internal consistency for total scale and the psychomotor reactions subscale were strong, reliabilities for somatic reactions and psychosocial reactions subscales were low [75]. Moreover, a Norwegian study demonstrated that the four most informative tool items explained 68% of the variance of the expert score with the psychosocial reactions subscale contributing little to the tool [76]. Despite evidence to support validity [49,75,76], there is indication of need for tool revision. Moreover, although clinicians report the tool manual is clear, in clinical testing nurses report the tool is difficult to score and interpret [75,76].

The Pain Assessment Checklist for Seniors with Severe Dementia (PAC-SLAC) [77], developed by a Canadian team, is a conceptually sound comprehensive checklist of pain behaviors that addresses all six pain behavioral categories included in the American Geriatrics Society guidelines. In preliminary testing the PACSLAC showed initial reliability and validity based on retrospective judgments. In recent prospective testing of a Dutch version of the tool, interrater and intrarater reliabilities were high [75]. The tool includes 60 behavioral items; however, nearly half the items were not observed in over 90% of the study subjects, suggesting need for item reduction. Moreover, although internal consistency for total tool score was good, results for subscale scores were poor to moderate, suggesting need for tool revision. PACSLAC also showed good construct and congruent validity and was rated the most preferred behavioral pain tool by Dutch nurses. The Dutch research team found the PACSLAC to be the most promising tool for further development [75].

The Pain Assessment Checklist for Seniors with Severe Dementia–Dutch-Revised [75] is a 24-item preliminary tool with three subscales derived from the original PACSLAC based on factor analysis. Internal consistencies of the total tool and revised subscales are good. Moreover, the reduced version of the scale correlated highly with the original tool suggesting validity is retained; however, further prospective, confirmatory testing in an independent sample is needed.

The Pain Assessment in Advanced Dementia (PAINAD) Scale [78] was developed as a short, easy to use observation tool for behavioral pain assessment in nonverbal older adults with advanced dementia. Originally developed in English, the PAINAD has been translated and tested in Italian [79], Dutch [75], and German [80]. Although interrater [75,78–80] and test-retest [75,79,80] reliability have been supported, internal consistency is only moderate with the breathing item scoring persistently low [75]. Evidence currently supports several types of validity. Despite mounting evidence of reliability and validity, however, issues persist. The PAINAD measures severity based on scoring of behaviors that has not been substantiated in the literature. Moreover, in clinical testing nurses report experiencing the PAINAD as too concise with too few pain cues included [75]. In one study, raters did not use the breathing item in painful situations in over 80% of participants with pain [75]. In another study nurses expressed uncertainty regarding the consolability item [80]. The limited number of items limits the ability of the PAINAD to detect pain in persons with dementia with more subtle behavioral presentation.

Behavioral Pain Scale (BPS) [81] is a French tool developed for critically ill sedated adult patients undergoing mechanical ventilation. Initial reports of tool testing in trauma and postoperative ICUs in France [81] and Morocco [82] seem to provide initial support for reliability and validity; however, results are largely based on total number of observations rather than individual patients. Initial validation studies were conducted with younger adults; testing in older adult populations is needed. An English version of the BPS was tested in Australia in unconscious medical and surgical ICU patients including some older patients (median age, 64 years; range, 16–82 years) [83]. Reported reliabilities were variable suggesting need for further testing under more tightly controlled conditions. Data were skewed toward the lower end of the BPS, which may indicate inaccurate scaling of items. Patients were not assessed for delirium in any of these three BPS studies. Further testing of the BPS is needed to establish reliability and validity using patients as the unit of analysis and, moreover, testing in older adults is needed.

Critical Care Pain Observation Tool (CPOT) [55] is a French tool developed by a Canadian team for assessment of pain behaviors in critically ill patients unable to communicate verbally. The CPOT measures pain intensity by behavioral observation, which has not been substantiated in the literature. Initial tool testing was conducted in cognitively intact adult surgical patients with no delirium while unconscious, conscious and intubated, and following extubation. Internal consistency was not reported and interrater reliability was only moderate; further testing is necessary to establish reliability. Initial tool validity was supported. Although this tool shows promise, tool testing in critically ill older adult samples and testing in English-speaking populations are needed.

Summary

Pain is an important health problem for nonverbal older adults with dementia, delirium, and during episodes of severe critical illness requiring appropriate strategies for these vulnerable populations. A comprehensive approach to assessment is advocated including multiple sources of information to ensure a valid and reliable basis on which to make treatment decisions. Behavioral observation and surrogate report are essential components of a multifaceted approach to assessment that may include standardized behavioral pain tools. Although some currently available tools for behavioral assessment in nonverbal older adults show promise, there is currently no single tool with sufficient validity and reliability to warrant recommendation for broad adoption in clinical practice. Continued and concerted effort is needed to develop and validate tools for nonverbal populations.

References

[1] APS (American Pain Society). Principles of analgesic use in the treatment of acute pain and cancer pain. 5th edition. Glenview (IL): American Pain Society; 2003.

[2] AGS Panel on Persistent Pain in Older Persons. The management of persistent pain in older persons. J Am Geriatr Soc 2002;50:S205–24.

[3] Sakai KL. Language acquisition and brain development. Science 2005;310:815–9.

[4] Wimo A, Jonsson L, Winblad B. An estimate of the worldwide prevalence and direct costs of dementia in 2003. Dement Geriatr Cogn Disord 2006;21:175–81.

[5] American Psychiatric Association. Diagnostic and statistical manual of mental disorders: text revision edition: DSM-IV-TR. 4th edition. Washington DC: American Psychiatric Association; 2000.

[6] Hadjistavropoulos T, Herr K, Turk DC, et al. An interdisciplinary expert consensus statement on assessment of pain in older persons. Clin J Pain 2007;23:S1–43.

[7] Ferrell BA, Ferrell BR, Rivera L. Pain in cognitively impaired nursing home patients. J Pain Symptom Manage 1995;10:591–8.

[8] Fox PL, Raina P, Jadad AR. Prevalence and treatment of pain in older adults in nursing homes and other long-term care institutions: a systematic review. Can Med Assoc J 1999; 160:329–33.

[9] Proctor WR, Hirdes JP. Pain and cognitive status among nursing home residents in Canada. Pain Res Manag 2001;6:119–25.

[10] Blair M, Marczinski CA, Davis-Faroque N, et al. A longitudinal study of language decline in Alzheimer's disease and frontotemporal dementia. J Int Neuropsychol Soc 2007;13: 237–45.

[11] Vuorinen E, Laine M, Rinne J. Common pattern of language impairment in vascular dementia and in Alzheimer disease. Alzheimer Dis Assoc Disord 2000;14:81–6.

[12] Scherder EJ, Sergeant JA, Swaab DF. Pain processing in dementia and its relation to neuropathology. Lancet Neurol 2003;2:677–86.

[13] Scherder E, Bouma A, Borkent M, et al. Alzheimer patients report less pain intensity and pain affect than non-demented elderly. Psychiatry 1999;62:265–72.

[14] Benedetti F, Arduino C, Vighetti S, et al. Pain reactivity in Alzheimer patients with different degrees of cognitive impairment and brain electrical activity deterioration. Pain 2004;111: 22–9.

[15] Scherder E, Oosterman J, Swaab D, et al. Recent developments in pain in dementia. Br Med J 2005;330:461–4.

[16] Parmelee PA, Smith B, Katz IR. Pain complaints and cognitive status among elderly institution residents. J Am Geriatr Soc 1993;41:517–22.

[17] Nygaard HA, Jarland M. Are nursing home patients with dementia diagnosis at increased risk for inadequate pain treatment? Int J Geriatr Psychiatry 2005;20:730–7.

[18] Feldt KS, Ryden MB, Miles S. Treatment of pain in cognitively impaired compared with cognitively intact older patients with hip-fracture. J Am Geriatr Soc 1998;46:1079–85.

[19] Morrison RS, Siu AL. A comparison of pain and its treatment in advanced dementia and cognitively intact patients with hip fracture. J Pain Symptom Manage 2000;19:240–8.

[20] Williams CS, Zimmerman S, Sloane PD, et al. Characteristics associated with pain in long-term care residents with dementia. Gerontologist 2005;45:68–73.

[21] Wu N, Miller SC, Lapane K, et al. Impact of cognitive function on assessments of nursing home residents' pain. Med Care 2005;43:934–9.

[22] Horgas AL, Tsai P. Analgesic drug prescription and use in cognitively impaired nursing home residents. Nurs Res 1998;47:235–42.

[23] Bernabei R, Gambassi G, Lapane K, et al. Management of pain in elderly patients with cancer. JAMA 1998;279:1877–82.

[24] Agency for Health Care Policy and Research. Hospital inpatient statistics 1996. Washington, DC: US Department of Health and Human Services; 1999.

[25] McNicoll L, Pisani MA, Zhang Y, et al. Delirium in the intensive care unit: occurrence and clinical course in older patients. J Am Geriatr Soc 2003;51:591–8.

[26] Goy E, Ganzini L. Delirium, anxiety, and depression. In: Morrison RS, Meier DE, editors. Geriatric palliative care. New York: Oxford University Press; 2003. p. 286–303.

[27] Culp KR, Wakefield B, Dyck MJ, et al. Bioelectrical impedance analysis and other hydration parameters as risk factors for delirium in rural nursing home residents. J Gerontol A Biol Sci Med Sci 2004;59:813–7.

[28] Lipowski ZJ. Delirium: acute confusional states. New York: Oxford University Press; 1990.

[29] Inouye SK, Charpentier PA. Precipitating factors for delirium in hospitalized elderly persons: predictive model and interrelationship with baseline vulnerability. JAMA 1996;275:852–7.

[30] Young J, Inouye SK. Delirium in older people. BMJ 2007;334:842–6.

[31] Morrison RS, Magaziner J, Gilbert M, et al. Relationship between pain and opioid analgesics on the development of delirium following hip fracture. J Gerontol A Biol Sci Med Sci 2003;58:76–81.

[32] Schor JD, Levkoff SE, Lipsitz LA, et al. Risk factors for delirium in hospitalized elderly. JAMA 1992;267:827–31.

[33] Duggleby W, Lander J. Cognitive status and postoperative pain: older adults. J Pain Symptom Manage 1994;9:19–27.

[34] Lynch EP, Lazor MA, Gellis JE, et al. The impact of postoperative pain on the development of postoperative delirium. Anesth Analg 1998;86:781–5.

[35] Marcantonio ER, Juarez G, Goldman L, et al. The relationship of postoperative delirium with psychoactive medications. JAMA 1994;272:1518–22.

[36] Liptzin B, Levkoff SE. An empirical study of delirium subtypes. Br J Psychiatry 1992;161: 843–5.

[37] Albert MS, Levkoff SE, Reilly C, et al. The delirium symptom interview: an interview for the detection of delirium symptoms in hospitalized patients. J Geriatr Psychiatry Neurol 1992;5: 14–21.

[38] Bruera E, Fainsinger RL, Miller MJ, et al. The assessment of pain intensity in patients with cognitive failure: a preliminary report. J Pain Symptom Manage 1992;7:267–70.

[39] Decker SA, Perry AG. The development and testing of the PATCOA to assess pain in confused older adults. Pain Manag Nurs 2003;4:77–86.

[40] Angus DC, Kelley MA, Schmitz RJ, et al. Caring for the critically ill patient. Current and projected workforce requirements for care of the critically ill and patients with pulmonary disease: can we meet the requirements of an aging population? JAMA 2000;284:2762–70.

[41] Nelson JE, Meier DE, Oei EJ, et al. Self-reported symptom experience of critically ill cancer patients receiving intensive care. Crit Care Med 2001;29:277–82.

[42] Rotondi AJ, Chelluri L, Sirio C, et al. Patients' recollections of stressful experiences while receiving prolonged mechanical ventilation in an intensive care unit. Crit Care Med 2002; 30:746–52.

[43] Pennock BE, Crawshaw L, Maher T, et al. Distressful events in the ICU as perceived by patients recovering from coronary artery bypass surgery. Heart Lung 1994;23:323–7.

[44] Puntillo KA, Morris AB, Thompson CL, et al. Pain behaviors observed during six common procedures: results from Thunder project II. Crit Care Med 2004;32:421–7.

[45] Puntillo KA, White C, Morris AB, et al. Patients' perceptions and responses to procedural pain: results from Thunder project II. Am J Crit Care 2001;10:238–51.

[46] Jacobi J, Fraser G, Coursin DB, et al. Clinical practice guidelines for the sustained use of sedatives and analgesics in the critically ill adult. Crit Care Med 2002;30:119–41.

[47] Herr K, Coyne PJ, Key T, et al. Pain assessment in the nonverbal patient: position statement with clinical practice recommendations. Pain Manag Nurs 2006;7:44–52.

[48] Closs SJ, Barr B, Briggs M, et al. A comparison of five pain assessment scales for nursing home residents with varying degrees of cognitive impairment. J Pain Symptom Manage 2004;27:196–205.

[49] Pautex S, Herrmann F, Le Lous P, et al. Feasibility and reliability of four pain self-assessment scales and correlation with an observational rating scale in hospitalized elderly demented patients. J Gerontol A Biol Sci Med Sci 2005;60:524–9.

[50] Pautex S, Michon A, Guedira M, et al. Pain in severe dementia: self-assessment or observational scales? J Am Geriatr Soc 2006;54:1040–5.

[51] Buffum MD, Miaskowski C, Sands L, et al. A pilot study of the relationship between discomfort and agitation in patients with dementia. Geriatr Nurs 2001;22:80–5.

[52] Herr K, Garand L. Assessment and measurement of pain in older adults. Clin Geriatr Med 2001;17:457–78.

[53] Herr K, Bjoro K, Decker S. Tools for assessment of pain in nonverbal older adults with dementia: a state-of-the-science review. J Pain Symptom Manage 2006;31:170–92.

[54] Feldt KS. The Checklist of Nonverbal Pain Indicators (CNPI). Pain Manag Nurs 2000;1: 13–21.

[55] Gelinas C, Fillion L, Puntillo KA, et al. Validation of the critical-care pain observation tool in adult patients. Am J Crit Care 2006;15:420–7.

[56] Hurley AC, Volicer BJ, Hanrahan PA, et al. Assessment of discomfort in advanced Alzheimer patients. Res Nurs Health 1992;15:369–77.

[57] Pasero C, McCaffery M. Pain in the critically ill. Am J Nurs 2002;102:59–60.

[58] McCaffery M, Pasero C. Pain: clinical manual. 2nd edition. St. Louis (MO): Mosby; 1999.

[59] Bell ML. Postoperative pain management for the cognitively impaired older adult. Semin Perioper Nurs 1997;6:37–41.

[60] Hadjistavropoulos T, LaChapelle DL, MacLeod FK, et al. Measuring movement-exacerbated pain in cognitively impaired frail elders. Clin J Pain 2000;16:54–63.

[61] Mentes JC, Teer J, Cadogan MP. The pain experience of cognitively impaired nursing home residents: perceptions of family members and certified nursing assistants. Pain Manag Nurs 2004;5:118–25.

[62] Nygaard HA, Jarland M. Chronic pain in nursing home residents: patients' self-report and nurses' assessment. Tidsskr Nor Laegeforen 2005;125:1349–51.

[63] Kovach CR, Weissman DE, Griffie J, et al. Assessment and treatment of discomfort for people with late-stage dementia. J Pain Symptom Manage 1999;18:412–9.

[64] Buffum MD, Sands L, Miaskowski C, et al. A clinical trial of the effectiveness of regularly scheduled versus as-needed administration of acetaminophen in the management of discomfort in older adults with dementia. J Am Geriatr Soc 2004;52:1093–7.

[65] Manfredi PL, Breuer B, Wallenstein S, et al. Opioid treatment for agitation in patients with advanced dementia. Int J Geriatr Psychiatry 2003;18:700–5.

[66] Chibnall JT, Tait RC, Harman B, et al. Effect of acetaminophen on behavior, well-being, and psychotropic medication use in nursing home residents with moderate-to-severe dementia. J Am Geriatr Soc 2005;53:1921–9.

[67] Kovach CR, Noonan PE, Griffie J, et al. Use of the assessment of discomfort in dementia protocol. Appl Nurs Res 2001;14:193–200.

[68] Kovach CR, Noonan PE, Schlidt AM, et al. The Serial Trial Intervention: an innovative approach to meeting needs of individuals with dementia. J Gerontol Nurs 2006;32:18–25.

[69] Hadjistavropoulos T. Assessing pain in older persons with severe limitations in ability to communicate. In: Gibson SJ, Weiner DK, editors. Pain in older persons. Seattle (WA): IASP Press; 2005. p. 135–51.

[70] Stolee P, Hillier LM, Esbaugh J, et al. Instruments for the assessment of pain in older persons with cognitive impairment. J Am Geriatr Soc 2005;53:319–26.

[71] Zwakhalen SM, Hamers JP, Abu-Saad HH, et al. Pain in elderly people with severe dementia: a systematic review of behavioural pain assessment tools. BMC Geriatr 2006;6:3. Available at: http://www.biomedcentral.com/1471-2318-6-3.

[72] van Herk R, van Dijk M, Baar FP, et al. Observation scales for pain assessment in older adults with cognitive impairments or communication difficulties. Nurs Res 2007;56:34–43.

[73] Nygaard HA, Jarland M. The Checklist of Nonverbal Pain Indicators (CNPI): testing of reliability and validity in Norwegian nursing homes. Age Ageing 2006;35:79–81.

[74] Lefebvre-Chapiro S. The Doloplus group. The Doloplus 2 scale: evaluating pain in the elderly. European Journal of Palliative Care 2001;8:191–4.

[75] Zwakhalen SM, Hamers JP, Berger MP. The psychometric quality and clinical usefulness of three pain assessment tools for elderly people with dementia. Pain 2006;126:210–20.

[76] Holen JC, Saltvedt I, Fayers PM, et al. The Norwegian Doloplus-2, a tool for behavioural pain assessment: translation and pilot-validation in nursing home patients with cognitive impairment. Palliat Med 2005;19:411–7.

[77] Fuchs-Lacelle S, Hadjistavropoulos T. Development and preliminary validation of the pain assessment checklist for seniors with limited ability to communicate (PACSLAC). Pain Manag Nurs 2004;5:37–49.

[78] Warden V, Hurley AC, Volicer L. Development and psychometric evaluation of the Pain Assessment in Advanced Dementia (PAINAD) scale. J Am Med Dir Assoc 2003;4:9–15.

[79] Costardi D, Rozzini L, Costanzi C, et al. The Italian version of the Pain Assessment in Advanced Dementia (PAINAD) scale. Arch Gerontol Geriatr 2007;44:175–80.

[80] Schuler MS, Becker S, Kaspar R, et al. Psychometric properties of the German Pain Assessment in Advanced Dementia Scale (PAINAD-G) in nursing home residents. J Am Med Dir Assoc 2007;8:388–95.

[81] Payen JF, Bru O, Bosson JL, et al. Assessing pain in critically ill sedated patients by using a behavioral pain scale. Crit Care Med 2001;29:2258–63.

[82] Aissaoui Y, Zeggwagh AA, Zekraoui A, et al. Validation of a behavioral pain scale in critically ill, sedated, and mechanically ventilated patients. Anesth Analg 2005;101:1470–6.

[83] Young J, Siffleet J, Nikoletti S, et al. Use of a behavioural pain scale to assess pain in ventilated, unconscious and/or sedated patients. Intensive Crit Care Nurs 2006;22:32–9.

[84] Manfredi PL, Breuer B, Meier DE, et al. Pain assessment in elderly patients with severe dementia. J Pain Symptom Manage 2003;25:48–52.

[85] Cohen-Mansfield J, Creedon M. Nursing staff members' perceptions of pain indicators in persons with severe dementia. Clin J Pain 2002;18:64–73.

[86] Cohen-Mansfield J, Lipson S. Pain in cognitively impaired nursing home residents: how well are physicians diagnosing it? J Am Geriatr Soc 2002;50:1039–44.

[87] Horgas AL, Dunn K. Pain in nursing home residents. comparison of residents' self-report and nursing assistants' perceptions. incongruencies exist in resident and caregiver reports of pain; therefore, pain management education is needed to prevent suffering. J Gerontol Nurs 2001;27:44–53.

[88] Cohen-Mansfield J. Nursing staff members' assessments of pain in cognitively impaired nursing home residents. Pain Manag Nurs 2005;6:68–75.

[89] Cohen-Mansfield J. Relatives' assessment of pain in cognitively impaired nursing home residents. J Pain Symptom Manage 2002;24:562–71.

[90] Pasero C, McCaffery M. No self-report means no pain-intensity rating. Am J Nurs 2005;105:50–3.

[91] Jones KR, Fink R, Hutt E, et al. Measuring pain intensity in nursing home residents. J Pain Symptom Manage 2005;30:519–27.

[92] Zwakhalen SMG, Hamers JPH, Berger MPF. Improving the clinical usefulness of a behavioural pain scale for older people with dementia. J Adv Nurs 2007;58:493–502.

[93] Lane P, Kuntupis M, MacDonald S, et al. A pain assessment tool for people with advanced Alzheimer's and other progressive dementias. Home Healthc Nurse 2003;21:32–7.

[94] Basler HD, Huger D, Kunz R, et al. Assessment of pain in advanced dementia. Construct validity of the German PAINAD. Schmerz 2006;20:519–26.

[95] Leong IY, Chong MS, Gibson SJ. The use of a self-reported pain measure, a nurse-reported pain measure and the PAINAD in nursing home residents with moderate and severe dementia: a validation study. Age Ageing 2006;35:252–6.

[96] Leong IY, Nuo TH. Prevalence of pain in nursing home residents with different cognitive and communicative abilities. Clin J Pain 2007;23:119–27.

ELSEVIER
SAUNDERS

CLINICS IN
GERIATRIC
MEDICINE

Clin Geriatr Med 24 (2008) 263–274

Special Issues and Concerns in the Evaluation of Older Adults Who Have Pain

Kenneth L. Kirsh, PhD[a], Howard S. Smith, MD[b],*

[a]*Pharmacy Practice and Science, University of Kentucky,*
725 Rose Street, 201B, Lexington, KY 40536–0082, USA
[b]*Department of Anesthesiology, Albany Medical College,*
47 New Scotland Avenue, MC-131, Albany, NY 12208, USA

Nearly all persons, including older adults, experience moderate to severe acute pain at some time during the course of their lives. This is most often in association with surgical procedures, medical conditions, or physical trauma. Untreated acute pain has been shown to prolong hospital stays and increase medical costs [1,2] and may initiate progression to chronic pain [3–5] and unnecessary suffering. When it comes to chronic pain, studies find that 10% to 55% of persons in the general population report significant current chronic pain. Chronic pain decreases quality of life [6], decreases work productivity, and markedly increases societal costs [7,8]. It has been estimated that the overall economic burden of untreated pain in the United States is more than 100 billion dollars per year in the United States [9].

Given that pain is an important and costly issue, dealing with the evaluation of the older adult who has pain presents unique challenges. From a paternal standpoint, we might assume that older patients are not susceptible to problems of abuse and addiction. We might fear upsetting patients by asking pointed questions and being perceived as inappropriate. Further, we might be worried about scaring patients away from treatment modalities, such as opioids, by pursuing such questions. Indeed, there is a subset of elderly patients who have pain and have fears about addiction and need to be convinced to try these medications. The potential exists that we might "scare off" this group that might otherwise benefit from aggressive pain management.

---

* Corresponding author.
E-mail address: smithh@mail.amc.edu (H.S. Smith).

0749-0690/08/$ - see front matter © 2008 Elsevier Inc. All rights reserved.
doi:10.1016/j.cger.2007.12.005

On the other side of the argument, addiction and abuse issues are no longer the sole purview of the young. Prescription drug abuse is increasing in
our country, and it knows no predefined age limits. We owe due diligence
to this problem by pursuing proper assessment and documentation for all
patients, regardless of age. Thus, the balancing act begins between educating
our fearful patients that they are not likely to become addicted without
a strong genetic vulnerability while also monitoring for those cases that
may be difficult to manage.

Prevalence of substance use problems in pain populations

The prevalence of substance use disorders is significantly higher in many
medical populations as compared with the normal population, with studies
identifying current substance use disorders in 19% to 26% of hospitalized
populations [10,11], 40% to 60% of persons sustaining major trauma [12],
and 5% to 67% of persons treated for depression [13]. Because such medical
populations are at high risk for experiencing acute and chronic pain, a relatively high prevalence of substance use problems is expected in persons
treated for pain, regardless of their age. Conversely, pain is identified at relatively high rates in populations seeking treatment for addictive disease. A
recent study found that chronic severe pain was experienced by 37% of
methadone maintenance patients and 24% of inpatients admitted for treatment of addiction, whereas pain of any type or duration during the past
week was reported by 80% of methadone maintenance patients and 78%
of inpatients [14]. Thus, older patients, who are more likely to have a medical
condition, should be evaluated carefully for aspects of substance misuse or
abuse. In addition, those older adults who have a known history of past
substance abuse, combined with current pain issues, need to be carefully
assessed and monitored.

With the aforementioned higher prevalence of substance use disorders in
the medically ill, combined with a general fear of overprescribing controlled
substances, such as opioids, the potential exists for older patients to be
denied access to the pain care they might need. Indeed, despite the fact
that national guidelines exist for the treatment of pain disorders, such as
cancer, pain continues to be undertreated [15–17]. In one advanced disease
type, cancer, it has been reported that approximately 40% to 50% of
patients who have metastatic disease and 90% of patients who have
terminal cancer or other advanced diseases experience unrelieved pain
[15–17]. Furthermore, inadequate treatment of cancer pain is even a greater
possibility if the patient is a member of an ethnic minority, female, elderly,
a child, or a substance abuser [18]. Thus, in pain treatment, we sometimes
have conflicting multiple biases that can lead to poor management, mutual
suspicion and alienation, and suffering for patients unless these biases are
adequately addressed.

Substance abuse in hospice, an exemplar of potential problems in older adults

Because pain management is an essential aspect of the palliative care of the dying patient and denying dying patients adequate analgesia is not accepted practice, discussion of these patients provides perhaps the best overview of the challenges faced when evaluating and treating chronic pain in the older patient [19]. Across the United States, hospice organizations have taken an active role in reducing pain and improving the quality of life of dying people. For most patients receiving hospice care, pain management proceeds in an uneventful fashion when issues of drug addiction or diversion are concerned. In some cases, however, when patients or their family members have preexisting substance abuse problems, management becomes more difficult and complex. Hospice nurses struggle disproportionately with this small percentage of patients. Given the high prevalence of addiction in our society in general and the rising tide of prescription drug abuse and diversion in particular, hospice nurses responsible for case management must be attentive to signs indicating problems with substance abuse or drug diversion in their cases and develop case management strategies for coping with these challenges.

Aggressive treatment of pain in hospice patients is sometimes hampered by misplaced fears of addiction. These fears are the primary patient and family-related barriers to pain management [17]. Although most fears of addiction are misplaced, in some patients and families, a history of drug or alcohol abuse makes these concerns a reality. Addiction is a common problem in our society, and prescription drug abuse has been increasing [20]. Aggressive pain management in hospice patients can sometimes be complicated by the presence of addiction in the patient or family members, and although there are relatively few such cases, they are labor-intensive and emotionally draining and raise difficult clinical and ethical dilemmas. This issue has been the subject of little empiric study, although clinical experience suggests it is no less common than one might expect based on the norms of drug abuse in the population at large.

In the small number of empiric studies related to this issue, substance abuse and misuse among patients admitted to hospice care units are not uncommon and are often missed in initial assessments and longer term follow-up. A survey conducted by Bruera and colleagues [21] found that more than 25% of patients who had cancer and were admitted to a palliative care unit had a problem with alcohol abuse. Only one third of the patients with alcohol abuse had a documented diagnosis of alcoholism in their charts, however, even though all these patients had undergone numerous hospital admissions and medical interventions. Estimates are that 6% to 15% of the general population in the United States has a substance abuse problem [22–24]; hence, it is reasonable that some portion of this 6% to 15% is also reflected in the makeup of patients entering hospice care. Other hospice patients may develop psychiatric conditions related to end-of-life issues, and still other hospice patients have preexisting psychiatric disorders. These patients may also be at increased risk for abusing and misusing prescribed medications. Such patients have been referred to as so-called "chemical copers" [21], and their patterns of drug use are problematic at times, leading to overmedication and poor outcomes.

There is little doubt that substance abuse–related issues make case management more difficult. Adequate pain control is more difficult to obtain and maintain when patients are abusing substances [25]. In addition, families with substance abuse problems tend to have poorer coping skills and more chaotic home environments than families without these problems [26,27]. To complicate the situation further, hospice care involves more than the identified patient. Friends and family members are also intimately involved in end-of-life care and also have the opportunity to engage in misuse or diversion of the patient's prescribed medication. Because hospice care occurs within the context of the family and community, chaotic dysfunctional family behavior can have a serious impact on patient management. Some dying patients have family members who are substance abusers, who are psychiatrically ill, and who have criminal histories.

Unchecked substance abuse perpetuates a dying patient's suffering, also complicating symptom management, impeding diagnosis and treatment of psychiatric problems, and creating tension for an already fragile social support network of family and caregivers [28]. Counseling, medication, and pain and symptom management techniques that are not beyond the scope of routine clinical practice can be used successfully to provide supportive care that patients and their caregivers need to allow for desired outcomes in end-of-life care.

Some clinicians and nurses fail to appreciate the deleterious impact of addiction on palliative care efforts, whereas others view addiction as an intractable problem for which interventions are likely to fail in any case. Furthermore, some of these clinicians may believe that not only is it impossible to decrease a patient's use of alcohol or illicit substance successfully while in palliative care but erroneously believe that such a decrease is tantamount to depriving a dying patient of a source of pleasure [28]. In fact, chemically dependent patients spend little of their time high or euphoric, even when engaging in substance use. Instead, most of their time is spent feeling depressed, isolated, and withdrawn or engaging in behaviors they themselves consider to be demeaning or degrading, particularly those related to drug procurement. Indeed, what is so mystifying about addiction is the tenacity of behaviors that are so infrequently and inconsistently rewarded. The typical mental state of the chemically dependent individual is rarely one of euphoria; instead, it is more often a global state of unpleasantness, boredom, and loneliness. This suffering is no less a legitimate target of hospice intervention than any other form simply because it is at the patient's (or family's) own hand. The nihilism that sometimes characterizes the approach to this problem can simply lead to more unchecked abuse-related behavior and a perpetuation of suffering.

Anecdotal evidence suggests that diversion occurs in at least some hospice cases [29,30], but there are no empiric studies on this issue. Pain medications can be diverted for several reasons. Some family members may have a preexisting substance abuse disorder and may abuse the medication prescribed to the patient for pain relief. Some anecdotal evidence suggests that family members or caregivers may use the patient's pain medication to deal with the stress of coping with the illness. In other situations, the patient or the patient's family may divert the drugs by selling them or allowing them to be sold on the street to provide funds for basic needs. Until basic data on drug diversion associated with hospice patients are gathered, the severity and the scope of the problem remain unknown.

The relative monetary value of prescription drugs is also an unavoidable issue. Diversion of prescription drugs can provide patients and their families with extra funds at a stressful time. Monies obtained through illicit sales of prescription drugs can improve patient quality of life by providing needed goods and services that might be otherwise unavailable or by allowing the patient or the family access to luxuries typically inaccessible to them. Unfortunately, because of the widespread problem of addiction and prescription drug abuse, pain medications typically prescribed to hospice patients are easily converted to cash in most communities in the United States. Pain medications may represent unexpected resources that some patients and families are unable to resist exploiting. The phenomenon of the "patient dealer," new in drug abuse and diversion circles over the past few years, has been noted to have begun in Maine with the case of a woman who had advanced cancer selling her medications [31].

Need for good documentation

Some experts suggest that when opioids are required as a component of chronic pain treatment, a set of universal precautions be used in managing all patients. This is based on the understanding that similar to the paradigm of universal precautions followed in infectious disease settings, the risk for an individual patient to misuse opioids cannot be reliably predicted and the misuse of opioids has potentially seriously negative consequences for the patient and the prescriber. In addition, application of precautions only to selected patients risks stigmatizing those patients. Therefore, it is argued that all patients receive careful assessment with formulation of a differential diagnosis of pain; appropriate assessment of psychologic and substance use issues; informed consent for treatment; clear treatment agreement; a trial of treatment with clear goals; assessment and periodic reassessment of pain level [32], function, and salient other issues; and good documentation of care.

When considering the content of chart notes in the pain management of the older adult, there may be a tendency to gloss over or shy away from sensitive areas of inquiry for fear of embarrassing the patient or discussing something that is not likely to occur. According to model guidelines for opioid therapy developed by the Federation of State Medical Boards, however, the medical record should document the nature and intensity of the pain, current and past treatments for pain, underlying or coexisting diseases or conditions, the effect of the pain on physical and psychologic function, and history of substance abuse [33]. No distinctions are made for sensitive areas, such as substance abuse, simply based on the demographic profile of the patient. To assess the appropriateness, course, and outcome of therapy, information should be available concerning the patient evaluation, treatment plan, informed consent and agreement for treatment, monitoring approach, consultation requests, medical record keeping, and compliance with the controlled substances laws and regulations [33]. Recent standards promulgated by the Joint Commission on the Accreditation of Health Care Organizations also recommend that physicians record the results of their pain assessment in a way that facilitates regular reassessment and follow-up [34].

Physicians who adequately assess patients before and during opioid therapy may still encounter problems as a result of poor documentation. For example, in a chart review of 300 patients who had chronic pain, 61% had no documentation of a treatment plan [35]. Similarly, a review of the initial consultation notes of 513 patients who had acute musculoskeletal pain revealed that only 43% of historical findings and 28% of physical examination findings were documented [36]. In a review of 520 randomly selected visits at an outpatient oncology practice, quantitative assessment of pain scores was virtually absent ($<1\%$) and qualitative assessment of pain occurred in only 60% of cases [37]. Finally, a review of medical records of 111 randomly selected patients who underwent urine toxicology screens in a cancer center found that documentation was infrequent: 37.8% of physicians failed to list a reason for the test, and 89% of the charts did not include the results of the test [38].

Domains of interest for documentation

Risk screening

Standard assessment of substance use history, when performed in medical settings, most often includes inquiry about past and present alcohol, tobacco, and street drug use, including treatment, and screening with common instruments, such as the CAGE or the drug abuse screening test (DAST) [39,40]. Several screens specifically aimed at assessing risk for medication misuse in the pain treatment setting are in evolution [41,42]. One promising screen is the Screener and Opioid Assessment for

Patients in Pain (SOAPP), which has been validated as a 14- and 20-question screen and is now undergoing testing in a shorter form [43]. Another is the Opioid Risk Tool (ORT), a 5-question screen that is easily used in a pain treatment setting and discriminates well between high- and low-risk patients [44].

When considering how to incorporate the aforementioned content areas in chart notes on an ongoing basis after the initial screening, it is important to consider four main domains in assessing pain outcomes for those older patients being maintained on an opioid regimen: (1) pain relief, (2) functional outcomes, (3) side effects, and (4) drug-related behaviors. These domains have been labeled the "Four A's" (analgesia, activities of daily living, adverse effects, and aberrant drug-related behaviors) for teaching purposes [45]. There are, of course, many different ways to think about these domains, and multiple attempts to capture them are discussed here.

Pain Assessment and Documentation Tool

The Pain Assessment and Documentation Tool (PADT), based on the Four A's mentioned previously, is a simple charting device that is intended to focus on key outcomes and provide a consistent way to document progress in pain management therapy over time. Twenty-seven clinicians completed the preliminary version of the PADT for 388 opioid-treated patients [46,47]. The PADT is a brief two-sided chart note that can be readily included in the patient's medical record. It was designed to be intuitive, pragmatic, and adaptable to clinical situations. In the field trial, it took clinicians between 10 and 20 minutes to complete the tool.

By addressing the need for documentation, the PADT can assist clinicians in meeting their obligations for ongoing assessment and documentation. Although the PADT is not intended to replace a progress note, it is well suited to complement existing documentation with a focused evaluation of outcomes that are clinically relevant and address the need for evidence of appropriate monitoring.

The decision to assess the four domains subsumed under the shorthand designation, the Four A's, was based on clinical experience, the positive comments received by the investigators during educational programs on opioid pharmacotherapy for nonmalignant pain, and an evolving national movement that recognizes the need to approach opioid therapy with a "balanced" response. This response recognizes the legitimate need to provide optimal therapy to appropriate patients and the need to acknowledge the potential for abuse, diversion, and addiction [45]. The value of assessing pain relief, side effects, and aspects of functioning has been emphasized repeatedly in the literature [35,48–51]. Documentation of drug-related behaviors is a relatively new concept that is being explored for the first time in the PADT.

Defining abuse and addiction in the older patient with pain

When assessing drug-taking behaviors in the older patient with pain using the methods described previously, issues exist that increase the difficulty in arriving at a diagnosis of abuse or addiction. These issues include the problem of undertreatment of pain, sociocultural influences on the definition of aberrancy in drug taking, and the importance of illness-related variables [52,53].

Whereas abuse is defined as the use of an illicit drug or a prescription drug without medical indication, addiction refers to the continued use of either type of drug in a compulsive manner regardless of harm to the user or others. When a drug is prescribed for a medically diagnosed purpose, however, less assuredness exists as to the behaviors that could be deemed aberrant, and the potential for a diagnosis of drug abuse or addiction increases. Although it is difficult to disagree with the aberrancy of certain behaviors, such as intravenous injection of oral formulations, various other behaviors are less blatant, such as a patient who is experiencing unrelieved pain taking an extra dose of prescribed opioids [52,53].

The ability to categorize these questionable behaviors as apart from the social or cultural norm is also based on the assumption that certain parameters of normative behavior exist. Although it is useful to consider the degree of aberrancy of a given behavior, recognizing that these behaviors exist along a continuum with certain behaviors being less aberrant (eg, aggressively requesting medication), whereas other behaviors are more aberrant (eg, injection of oral formulations), in the area of prescription drug use, empiric data defining these parameters do not exist. If a large portion of patients were found to engage in a certain behavior, it might be normative and judgments regarding aberrancy should be influenced accordingly [52,53].

A differential diagnosis should also be considered if questionable behaviors occur during pain treatment. A true addiction (substance dependence) is only one of many possible interpretations. A diagnosis of pseudoaddiction should also be taken into account if the patient is reporting distress associated with unrelieved symptoms. Impulsive drug use may also be indicative of another psychiatric disorder, diagnosis of which may have therapeutic implications. On occasion, aberrant drug-related behaviors seem to be causally related to a mild encephalopathy, with perplexity concerning the appropriate therapeutic regimen. On rare occasions, questionable behaviors imply criminal intent. These diagnoses are not mutually exclusive [52,53].

Varied and repeated observations over time may be necessary to categorize questionable behaviors properly. Perceptive psychiatric assessment is crucial and may require evaluation by consultants who can elucidate the complex interactions among personality factors and psychiatric illness. Some older patients may be self-medicating symptoms of anxiety or depression, insomnia, or problems of adjustment (eg, boredom attributable to decreased ability to engage in usual activities and hobbies). Others may have character pathologic conditions that may be the more prominent determinant of drug-taking behavior. Patients who have borderline personality disorders, for example, may use prescription medications in an impulsive manner that regulates inner tension; expresses anger at physicians, friends, or family; or improves chronic emptiness of boredom. Psychiatric assessment is vitally important for the population without a prior history of substance abuse and the population of known substance abusers who have a high incidence of psychiatric comorbidity [54].

Using the results of ongoing evaluation

Simply broaching the sensitive topic of drug abuse with older patients with pain is not enough. Once the screening and ongoing assessments are completed, a plan must be made for those in whom problems are found. In short, some older patients with pain are best managed in a primary care setting; some in a primary care setting with support from specialists; and some by a specialist with specific skills in an area of need, such as a pain specialist, addiction specialist, or psychiatrist [32]. There are advantages and disadvantages to each setting. Primary care providers tend to have broader and more longitudinal knowledge of the patient and are in a better position to integrate care of pain with care of other medical issues. Specialists tend to have more depth of knowledge and expertise in management of a particular aspect of the patient's medical issues and may provide better care when a particular problem is prominent, such as addiction or psychiatric instability. Many variables may contribute to determination of the best setting of care for an individual patient. No formula can dictate which professional should manage a particular clinical pain problem, but consideration of several variables may be helpful in decision making. The most appropriate management setting for a patient may change as his or her presentation changes.

Summary

It is important to realize that issues of abuse and addiction exist and are problematic for everyone involved in health care and that it is no longer simply a problem of the young or recreational street users. Prescription drug abuse is growing in our country, and all patients need to be monitored carefully. If we approach pain management and addiction assessment from a universal guidelines approach, we may be successful in treating all our older patients equally while also broaching sensitive topic areas that may have been avoided for fear of impropriety in the past.

References

[1] Chelly JE, Ben-David B, Williams BA, et al. Anesthesia and postoperative analgesia: outcomes following orthopedic surgery. Orthopedics 2003;26(Suppl 8):S865–71.

[2] Skinner HB. Multimodal acute pain management. Am J Orthop 2004;33(Suppl 5):5–9.

[3] Carr DB, Goudas LC. Acute pain. Lancet 1999;353(9169):2051–8.

[4] Dahl JB, Møiniche S. Pre-emptive analgesia. Br Med Bull 2004;71:13–27.

[5] Young Casey C, Greenberg MA, Nicassio PM, et al. Transition from acute to chronic pain and disability: a model including cognitive, affective, and trauma factors. Pain 2008;134: 69–79.

[6] van der Waal JM, Terwee CB, van der Windt DA, et al. Health-related and overall quality of life of patients with chronic hip and knee complaints in general practice. Qual Life Res 2005; 14(3):795–803.

[7] Collins JJ, Baase CM, Sharda CE, et al. The assessment of chronic health conditions on work performance, absence, and total economic impact for employers. J Occup Environ Med 2005;47(6):547–57.

[8] McCarberg BH, Billington R. Consequences of neuropathic pain: quality-of-life issues and associated costs. Am J Manag Care 2006;12(Suppl 9):S263–8.

[9] Griffin RM. The price tag on pain. WebMD (C.G. Mathis, Reviewer.) Available at: http://men.webmd.com/features/price-tag-on-pain. Accessed May 25, 2007.

[10] Brems C, Johnson ME, Wells RS, et al. Rates and sequelae of the coexistence of substance use and other psychiatric disorders. Int J Circumpolar Health 2002;61(3):224–44.

[11] Passik SD, Kirsh KL, Donaghy KB, et al. Pain and aberrant drug-related behaviors in medically ill patients with and without histories of substance abuse. Clin J Pain 2006; 22(2):173–81.

[12] Norman SB, Tate SR, Anderson KG, et al. Do trauma history and PTSD symptoms influence addiction relapse context? Drug Alcohol Depend 2007;90:89–96.

[13] Sullivan MD, Edlund MJ, Steffick D, et al. Regular use of prescribed opioids: association with common psychiatric disorders. Pain 2005;119(1–3):95–103 [Epub 2005 Nov 17].

[14] Rosenblum A, Joseph H, Fong C, et al. Prevalence and characteristics of chronic pain among chemically dependent patients in methadone maintenance and residential treatment facilities. JAMA 2003;289(18):2370–8.

[15] Ramer L, Richardson JL, Cohen MZ, et al. Multimeasure pain assessment in an ethnically diverse group of patients with cancer. J Transcult Nurs 1999;10(2):94–101.

[16] Glajchen M, Fitzmartin RD, Blum D, et al. Psychosocial barriers to cancer pain relief. Cancer Pract 1995;3(2):76–82.

[17] Ward SE, Goldberg N, Miller-McCauley V, et al. Patient-related barriers to management of cancer pain. Pain 1993;52:319–24.

[18] Joranson DE, Gilson AM. Policy issues and imperatives in the use of opioids to treat pain in substance abusers. J Law Med Ethics 1994;22(3):215–23.

[19] Whitecar PS, Jonas AP, Clasen ME. Managing pain in the dying patient. Am Fam Physician 2000;61(3):755–64.

[20] SAMHSA. 1999 National Household Survey on Drug Abuse. Substance Abuse and Mental Health Services Administration (SAMHSA) Report Series; 1999.

[21] Bruera E, Moyano J, Seifert L, et al. The frequency of alcoholism among patients with pain due to terminal cancer. J Pain Symptom Manage 1995;10:599–604.

[22] Colliver JD, Kopstein AN. Trends in cocaine abuse reflected in emergency room episodes reported to DAWN. Public Health Rep 1991;106:59–68.

[23] Gfroerer J, Brodsky M. The incidence of illicit drug use in the United States, 1962–1989. Br J Addict 1992;87:1345–51.

[24] Regier DA, Farmer ME, Rae DS, et al. Comorbidity of mental disorders with alcohol and other drug abuse. JAMA 1990;264:2511–8.

[25] McCorquodale S, De Faye B, Bruera E. Palliative care rounds: case report: pain control in an alcoholic cancer patient. J Pain Symptom Manage 1993;8:177–80.
[26] Cook B, Winokur G. Alcoholism as a family dysfunction. Psychiatr Ann 1993;23:508–12.
[27] Mansky P. Reminiscence of an addictionologist: thoughts of a researcher and clinician. Psychiatr Q 1993;64:81–106.
[28] Passik SD, Theobald DE. Managing addiction in advanced cancer patients: why bother? J Pain Symptom Manage 2000;19:229–34.
[29] Scham M, Scham A. Hospices: medical and legal considerations. Leg Med 1985;297–322.
[30] Thornton ES, Burrow MA. Possible diversion of pain medication occurs in home hospice setting. Oncol Nurs Forum 1996;23:118.
[31] Hancock CM. OxyContin use and abuse. Clin J Oncol Nurs 2002;6(2):109.
[32] Gourlay D, Heit H. Universal precautions: a matter of mutual trust and responsibility. Pain Med 2006;7(2):210–1 author reply 212.
[33] Federation of State Medical Boards of United States, Inc. Model guidelines for the use of controlled substances for the treatment ofpain. 1998. Available at: http://www.fsmb.org. Accessed April 10, 2003.
[34] Phillips DM. JCAHO pain management standards are unveiled. Joint Commission on Accreditation of Healthcare Organizations. JAMA 2000;284:428–9.
[35] Clark JD. Chronic pain prevalence and analgesic prescribing in a general medical population. J Pain Symptom Manage 2002;23:131–7.
[36] Solomon DH, Schaffer JL, Katz JN, et al. Can history and physical examination be used as markers of quality? An analysis of the initial visit note in musculoskeletal care. Med Care 2000;38:383–91.
[37] Rhodes DJ, Koshy RC, Waterfield WC, et al. Feasibility of quantitative pain assessment in outpatient oncology practice. J Clin Oncol 2001;19:501–8.
[38] Passik SD, Schreiber J, Kirsh KL, et al. A chart review of the ordering and documentation of urine toxicology screens in a cancer center: do they influence patient management? J Pain Symptom Manage 2000;19:40–4.
[39] Brown RL, Rounds LA. Conjoint screening questionnaires for alcohol and other drug abuse: criterion validity in a primary care practice. Wis Med J 1995;94(3):135–40.
[40] Gavin DR, Ross HE, Skinner HA. Diagnostic validity of the drug abuse screening test in the assessment of DSM-III drug disorders. Br J Addict 1989;84(3):301–7.
[41] Akbik H, Butler SF, Budman SH, et al. Validation and clinical application of the Screener and Opioid Assessment for Patients with Pain (SOAPP). J Pain Symptom Manage 2006; 32(3):287–93.
[42] Friedman R, Li V, Mehrotra D. Treating pain patients at risk: evaluation of a screening tool in opioid-treated pain patients with and without addiction. Pain Med 2003;4(2):182–5.
[43] Butler SF, Budman SH, Fernandez K, et al. Validation of a screener and opioid assessment measure for patients with chronic pain. Pain 2004;112(1–2):65–75.
[44] Webster LR, Webster RM. Predicting aberrant behaviors in opioid-treated patients: preliminary validation of the Opioid Risk Tool. Pain Med 2005;6(6):432–42.
[45] Passik SD, Weinreb HJ. Managing chronic nonmalignant pain: overcoming obstacles to the use of opioids. Adv Ther 2000;17:70–83.
[46] Passik SD, Kirsh KL, Whitcomb LA, et al. A new tool to assess and document pain outcomes in chronic pain patients receiving opioid therapy. Clin Ther 2004;26(4):552–61.
[47] Passik SD, Kirsh KL, Whitcomb LA, et al. Monitoring outcomes during long-term opioid therapy for non-cancer pain: results with the Pain Assessment and Documentation Tool. J Opioid Manag 2005;1(5):257–66.
[48] Daut RL, Cleeland CS, Flanery RC. Development of the Wisconsin Brief Pain Questionnaire to assess pain in cancer and other diseases. Pain 1983;17:197–210.
[49] Cleeland CS, Ryan KM. Pain assessment: global use of the Brief Pain Inventory. Ann Acad Med Singap 1994;23:129–38.

[50] Melzack R. The McGill Pain Questionnaire: major properties and scoring methods. Pain 1975;1:277–99.

[51] McCarberg BH, Barkin RL. Long-acting opioids for chronic pain: pharmacotherapeutic opportunities to enhance compliance, quality of life, and analgesia. Am J Ther 2001;8: 181–6.

[52] Passik SD, Portenoy RK. Substance abuse issues in palliative care. In: Berger A, Portenoy R, Weissman D, editors. Principles and practice of supportive oncology. Philadelphia: Lippin-cott-Raven Publishers; 1998. p. 513–24.

[53] Passik SD, Portenoy RK, Ricketts PL. Substance abuse issues in cancer patients part 1: prevalence and diagnosis. Oncology 1998;12(4):517–21.

[54] Khantzian EJ, Treece C. DSM-III psychiatric diagnosis of narcotic addicts. Arch Gen Psychiatry 1985;42:1067–71.

ELSEVIER
SAUNDERS

CLINICS IN
GERIATRIC
MEDICINE

Clin Geriatr Med 24 (2008) 275–298

Pharmacotherapy of Pain in Older Adults

Scott A. Strassels, PharmD, PhD, BCPS[a,*],
Ewan McNicol, BSPharm, MS[b],
Rosy Suleman, PharmD[c]

[a]Division of Pharmacy Practice, University of Texas at Austin College of Pharmacy,
2409 University Avenue, PHR 3.208E, Austin, TX 78712, USA
[b]Tufts–New England Medical Center, 750 Washington Street Boston, MA 02111, USA
[c]Novartis Pharmaceuticals Corporation, 6250 Citricado Circle, Carlsbad, CA 92009, USA

Pain is a common reason for individuals to seek medical care. In 2003, three of the 20 most frequently mentioned reasons for outpatient department visits in the United States were related to stomach, head, or back pain [1]. Similarly, in a 1998 study, 21.5% of people in a multinational sample across Asia, Africa, Europe, and the Americas reported having pain most of the time during the previous 6 months [2]. More recently, a study of more than 46,000 European and Israeli people, the prevalence of chronic pain by country ranged from 12% to 30%, with a weighted average of 19% overall [3].

Pain is also an important occurrence among medical and surgical inpatients. In 2004, 45 million inpatient surgical procedures were performed in the United States [4]. Each person who undergoes surgery will have pain. Despite this reasonable expectation, biomedical evidence published during the past four decades indicates that pain is treated suboptimally for people in various patient populations, including medical and surgical inpatients, seriously ill hospitalized persons, minority and elderly persons who have cancer, and children at the end of life [5–13]. To further complicate matters, attempts to use diagnostic and demographic factors to predict which groups of people might be at lower risk for pain during hospitalization thus far have been unsuccessful [14].

Dr. Strassels has received research funding from excelleRx, Incorporated, and has served on advisory boards for Cephalon, King, Pricara, Ortho-McNeil, and Valeant Pharmaceuticals.
* Corresponding author.
E-mail address: scotts1@mail.utexas.edu (S.A. Strassels).

Important clinical, human, and economic consequences of this shortcoming include altered immune system functioning, diminished ability to function, increased risk of chronic pain, needless suffering, and higher health care costs [15–29]. One recent review estimated the prevalence of chronic pain to be about 50% among people who underwent thoracotomy, 30% to 81% of those who had a limb amputated, 11% to 51% of women who had breast surgery, up to 56% of people who underwent cholecystectomy, and up to 37% of people who had surgical repair of an inguinal hernia [24].

In the United States, 2002 costs of lost productive time caused by pain were estimated at $61.2 billion [25]. A sample of individuals who had neuropathic pain disorders incurred charges of more than $17,000 during calendar year 2000 compared with approximately $5715 in a matched control group without neuropathic pain [26]. In 2002, the costs of diabetes in the United States were estimated to be $132 billion, including $24.6 billion for chronic complications of this disease and $2.7 billion for neurologic symptoms, including pain [27]. A similar analysis of symptomatic diabetic peripheral neuropathy and its associated complications found that 2001 costs were approximately $237 million for neuropathy alone, but that costs soared to $10.9 billion when management of long-term complications were included [28]. In the United Kingdom, the average costs of adolescent chronic pain were estimated to be £8,027 per person, or approximately £3.8 billion in a year [29]. Although it is difficult to estimate the direct cost of acute postoperative pain, it is clear that pain may interfere with the ability to function in ways that are important to health care providers and patients and that this inability may contribute to longer stays in the hospital or to returning after discharge [18,23].

In the face of this large body of evidence indicating the need for significant improvement in pain management for many people, it is reasonable to ask why making lasting differences in the care of people with pain is so difficult. The challenges of pain management are related to the science and art of medical practice, and to an assortment of factors involving all levels of society and the health care system [30,31]. For example, in many professional medical, nursing, and pharmacy education curricula, education about pain and its treatment historically has been given little attention [32,33]. As a result, many health care providers lack a sufficient foundation in the clinical use of analgesics. This article seeks to help address that shortcoming, by providing a review of the pharmacotherapy of pain in older adults, with a focus on salicylates, nonsteroidal anti-inflammatory drugs (NSAIDs), and opioids.

Definitions

Before a useful discussion of this topic can be undertaken, it is important to ensure that a common lexicon is being used. The words used to define and describe pain are powerful and emotionally charged. They also often are used incorrectly or unclearly. A brief discussion of terms related to pain follows; the reader is referred to the International Association for the Study of Pain (IASP) for a more complete list.

Pain is a subjective, unpleasant, sensory, and emotional experience associated with actual or potential tissue damage, or described in terms of such damage [34]. More simply put, "pain is what the person says it is, existing whenever he says it does" [35]. The essence of these definitions is that pain is subjective, has multiple dimensions, without a clear relationship between the intensity of the sensation and tissue damage. Additionally, individuals may have pain even if communication is difficult or impossible. Furthermore, because pain is a subjective experience, it is critically important that patients' reports of pain be taken seriously [35].

Pain is described commonly in terms of its duration (eg, acute or chronic) and pathophysiology (eg, nociceptive or neuropathic) [36]. These constructs can be helpful by suggesting treatments that are likely to be effective, but they also can be misleading. For example, acute pain often is described as being of recent onset and limited duration, with a tendency to decrease over time, while chronic pain often is described as lasting for some undetermined, subjective period of time beyond that expected to be needed to heal [21]. Yet, acute pain from an injury may last much longer than expected, and the biochemical and cellular changes that accompany chronic pain may begin to appear relatively shortly after an injury [21].

Pathophysiology provides information that is often useful. Nociceptive pain refers to the result of noxious thermal, chemical, or mechanical stimuli that may damage normal tissue and can be delineated further into somatic or visceral subtypes [34,35]. Somatic pain originates in the skin, bones, muscle, and connective tissue, and usually is located specifically, while visceral pain originates in internal body structures and organs, and is located more generally. In contrast, neuropathic pain results from nervous system dysfunction of lesions on nerves, and may originate centrally or peripherally. Examples of central pain include phantom pain and sympathetically maintained processes, while peripherally originating neuropathic pain disorders include diabetic neuropathy and trigeminal neuralgia.

Dependence, tolerance, addiction, and pseudoaddiction

If a person on a drug develops a withdrawal syndrome when that substance is removed suddenly, the individual is physically dependent on that substance [37]. For opioid analgesics, the withdrawal syndrome generally includes signs of central arousal, such as insomnia, irritability, and agitation. Patients also may experience autonomic symptoms, including diarrhea, rhinorrhea, and sweating, as well as muscle spasms, gastrointestinal (GI) cramping, and other painful phenomena. Although typically associated with addiction, psychological dependence also may be an issue in appropriate pharmacotherapy. For instance, a person whose symptoms are relieved effectively by a drug or other intervention may be anxious about losing access to that intervention. The take-home message is that dependence is an expected physiologic response to use of some drugs, and is neither a sufficient nor a necessary aspect of addiction [37]. Although one often thinks of dependence relative to the opioid analgesics, this concept also applies to any other drug for which suddenly stopping use is discouraged. The best way to avoid development of a clinical withdrawal syndrome in a person thought to be dependent on a drug is to slowly decrease the dose.

Similarly, tolerance refers to the need for increased doses to produce a particular effect [37]. For a given drug, however, an individual may become tolerant to some effects, but not to others. For example, with the opioid analgesics, tolerance to sedation and respiratory effects typically develops quickly, while people generally develop tolerance to the constipating effects of these drugs slowly, if at all [38]. For this reason, a preventive bowel regimen is considered a routine part of therapy for individuals expected to be on opioid analgesics for an extended period of time.

Addiction is probably one of the most-misunderstood and feared phenomena associated with use of the opioid analgesics. This primary, chronic, neurobiological disease has genetic, psychosocial, and environmental dimensions [37]. As suggested by its multidimensional nature, it is also important to remember that while use of some drugs is associated with pleasurable effects, addiction is not only determined by the drug, but also by the user and the conditions in which use occurs. In general, however, addicted individuals may have impaired control over their drug use, use substances compulsively, continue to use despite harm, and crave the substance in question.

The fear that some health care providers have of prescribed analgesics leading to a patient to becoming addicted is an important contributor to the undertreatment of pain [39,40]. Among individuals who have acute pain, the biomedical evidence overwhelmingly indicates that the rate of iatrogenic addiction among people who do not have a history of substance abuse is vanishingly low [41–46]. The corresponding risk among people who have chronic pain remains incompletely understood, although in a recent in-depth discussion of this issue, Ballantyne and LaForge conclude that aberrant behaviors such as opioid drug-seeking and addiction occur frequently enough to be significantly concerning [47,48]. Although the clinical and legal importance of using clear, structured treatment plans and regular follow-up cannot be overemphasized in any person who has pain, the available evidence supports the contention that people who use opioid analgesics to relieve their pain on a mutually agreed upon schedule, without aberrant behaviors, and whose functioning and pain control are relatively stable, and who are willing to consider various treatment options are unlikely to become addicted [37]. Furthermore, although the risk of addiction cannot be ignored, particularly among people who are expected to need opioid analgesics for an extended period of time, neither should the large and compelling body of evidence indicating that the systematic undertreatment of pain—including use of subpotent analgesics, dosing regimens and routes that do not take full advantage of the pharmacokinetics and pharmacodynamics of the analgesic, and inappropriate reliance on as-needed use of these drugs—is common. Moreover, not only does the systematic undertreatment of pain unfairly penalize persons with pain, but it also can directly result in a phenomenon known as pseudoaddiction [49]. In this syndrome, the patient may (unsurprisingly) request analgesics before the next scheduled dose, doctor-shop, and act in other ways that are seen in people who abuse substances. The distinction is that when an undertreated individual's pain is treated appropriately, these aberrant behaviors disappear. Rather than waiting for a problem to develop, however, pseudoaddiction can be avoided by developing healthy trust between the patient and the health care team, using analgesics on a regular schedule, instead of on an as-needed basis, and use of adjuvants and nondrug treatments [49].

Clinically important age-related pharmacokinetic and pharmacodynamic changes

Pharmacokinetics refers to the effect of physiologic processes on drug disposition [50]. In general, the processes of most interest are absorption, distribution, metabolism, and excretion. Absorption is important in pain management, because the oral route of administration is preferred when it is available. Typically, however, the effect of age on passively absorbed drugs is thought to be small [51,52]. Drug distribution is a function of several parameters that can be affected by age, such as blood flow, binding of drugs to plasma proteins, and body fat percentage [52]. Of these, body fat percentage is thought to be the most clinically significant. This is because body fat tends to increase as a proportion of total body weight with increasing age, resulting in greater distribution for relatively lipophilic drugs, like fentanyl, and less-extensive distribution for comparatively hydrophilic drugs, such as morphine. In general, hepatic volume and blood flow decreases with age [52]. This phenomenon can result in decreased metabolism of drugs, and subsequently lower clearance and increased elimination half-life, although the effect of age on the cytochrome P450 system remains incompletely understood [52]. Renal function is thought to have important effects on drug elimination, and age-related decrements in glomerular function tend to occur. Drug and metabolite accumulation can occur in people whose renal function (generally estimated by creatinine clearance) is reduced, and who are taking drugs that are primarily renally excreted. In considering the pharmacotherapy of pain, the NSAIDs, and especially morphine (with its metabolites morphine-6-glucuronide and morphine-3-glucuronide), meperidine (with its metabolite, normeperidine), and propoxyphene (with its metabolite norpropoxyphene) are generally considered to be the most clinically important.

Pharmacodynamics refers to the clinical effects that result from use of a drug [50]. Age-related changes in these parameters are thought to be related to drug–receptor interactions and changes in homeostasis [52]. For example, the density of mu-opioid receptors, among others, generally declines with age. Similarly, older individuals tend to be more sensitive to some drugs, such as the benzodiazepines and opioids.

Choosing analgesics

There are many approaches to choosing the appropriate analgesic and dosing regimen for a given patient. One such pathway is to use a tool such as the World Health Organization three-step analgesic ladder, shown in Fig. 1 [53]. Originally designed to help clinicians caring for people with cancer pain, it also has been used by clinicians to guide the analgesic pharmacotherapy for other painful conditions. It is critically important to note that the ladder is merely a guide, and not intended to force clinicians and patients to use analgesics that are not appropriate for the patient or the individual's level of pain. For example, a person with newly diagnosed arthritis or early-stage cancer may have mild pain, and be well-suited by starting on the first step of the ladder and progressing as needed. In contrast, when

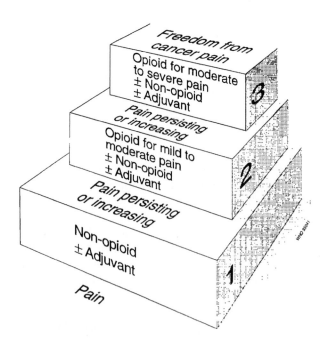

Fig. 1. The three-step analgesic ladder. (*Courtesy of* the World Health Organization; with permission).

a patient presents with moderate-to-severe pain, as with advanced disease or in the postoperative period, starting of the third step of the ladder is appropriate. Similarly, patients who have pain that waxes and wanes may need different level analgesics at different times, including no analgesic at some times. Use of this tool in this manner is also appropriate.

Salicylates

These drugs provide analgesic, antipyretic, anti-inflammatory, and antirheumatic activity [54]. Therapeutic serum concentrations of salicylate required to produce these effects differ widely, with substantially higher levels needed for anti-inflammatory activity than for antiplatelet, antipyretic, and analgesic effects. Aspirin is also well-known for its effects on platelet activity, although this topic is beyond the scope of this discussion. True salicylates (ie, aspirin and other salicylic acid derivatives) are converted to salicylic acid, while structurally-related compounds in this class (ie, diflunisal) that are not converted to salicylic acid are not considered to be true salicylates [54]. Pharmacologic distinctions aside, the drugs in this class have similar activity profiles, although aspirin inhibits prostaglandin synthesis more potently than other agents in this class. As a result, it has greater anti-inflammatory activity.

Salicylate absorption is complete and rapid after oral administration, although bioavailability is influenced by numerous factors, including the dosage form [54]. For example, absorption from rectal suppositories of these drugs is slower than from oral dosage forms. Absorbed drug is distributed widely, and excretion occurs by means of renal elimination. Salicylates are contraindicated in people who are hypersensitive to these drugs, NSAIDs, and tartrazine, also known as Food, Drug & Cosmetic yellow dye number 5. Aspirin-sensitive individuals are typically not cross-sensitive to sodium salicylate, salicylamide, and choline salicylate. Salicylates also may cause GI irritation and bleeding, and should be used cautiously in people who have a history of gastric or peptic ulcers. Salsalate and choline salicylate have been associated with less severe GI irritation than other salicylates [54].

Acetaminophen

Acetaminophen inhibits central prostaglandin synthesis with minimal inhibition of peripheral prostaglandin synthesis, without clinically significant reductions in inflammation, and adverse influences on gastric mucosa or platelet function [55]. It is absorbed rapidly, with peak plasma levels seen within 30 minutes to 1 hour, and is metabolized in the liver by conjugation and hydroxylation to inactive metabolites. Because of the risk of hepatotoxicity, acetaminophen should be used cautiously in patients who have liver disease, chronic alcoholism, and malnutrition, and the dosage should be limited to not more than 4000 mg per 24 hours in otherwise healthy adults, with lower limits in persons with diminished renal or hepatic function [55,56].

Although acetaminophen use is extremely common, recommended dosage limits often are overlooked. This is a potentially important problem, because many opioid analgesics are commercially available in fixed combinations with acetaminophen. Administering an opioid and acetaminophen separately allows the clinician more flexibility. In patients who receive acetaminophen rectally, clinicians should be aware that variability in rectal absorption may affect the dosage needed to provide analgesia for children [57,58]. It remains unclear if these results also apply to older adults who receive rectal acetaminophen, but clinicians should be aware of the potential for analgesia to be adversely affected in this way.

Nonsteroidal anti-inflammatory drugs

The body of literature regarding these drugs is vast, particularly regarding their effects on the cardiovascular system, and a full discussion of these issues is beyond the scope of this article. At present, there are 18 NSAIDs available in the United States [59]. These drugs reduce central and peripheral prostaglandin synthesis, but they do not inhibit the effects of prostaglandins already present, resulting in analgesia, followed by relatively delayed anti-inflammatory effects.

The NSAIDs have similar mechanisms of action and similar adverse effects, but there are differences in their potencies, time to onset of action, and duration of action, and responses may vary among patients [59]. As a result, inadequate pain relief from use of the dose maximum of one NSAID should not preclude switching to other drugs in this class.

NSAIDs are effective after various procedures, such as thoracotomy, major orthopedic, upper- and lower-abdominal, and minor outpatient surgery [60]. They also are used commonly for some painful chronic conditions, including osteoarthritis. The benefits of NSAIDs are particularly notable when they are used in combination with an opioid, and an opioid-sparing effect may result. Opioid adverse effects, such as sedation, nausea, and vomiting, are decreased in studies in which the combination was used. Additionally, the patient treated with NSAIDs in the perioperative period may be able to switch to an oral analgesic and return to a normal diet more rapidly [60].

NSAIDs cause important adverse effects that can limit their use. GI effects, including nausea, vomiting, and bleeding, are the most troublesome problems, and can result in death. Ketorolac generally has a low frequency of GI bleeding (if appropriately low doses are used), but the risk is increased when it is used in elderly patients who have a history of GI bleeding and when daily doses of over 120 mg are used for greater than 5 days [60]. Although there are some patients for whom NSAIDs are generally contraindicated (ie, solid organ transplant recipients), these drugs often are used postoperatively, and evidence generally indicates that the potential for clinical benefit outweighs the risk of postoperative bleeding.

Other adverse effects of NSAIDs include nephrotoxicity and hepatotoxicity [59,60]. NSAIDs are also highly protein bound, which can result in increased bioavailability of other highly bound drugs, including warfarin, methotrexate, digoxin, cyclosporine, oral antidiabetic agents, and anticonvulsants.

Cyclooxygenase-2 selective nonsteroidal anti-inflammatory drugs

Although cyclooxygenase (COX-2)selective NSAIDs are effective analgesics, their role in managing pain remains unclear, particularly in light of important safety questions that have led to the withdrawal of rofecoxib and valdecoxib from the United States market, leaving only celecoxib available. Aside from the current debate about the cardiovascular safety of the current generation of COX-2 selective NSAIDs, the primary short-term advantage of these drugs is the apparent lack of effect on platelet function. There are reports, however, of significantly increased international normalized ratios in people who were being treated with warfarin and rofecoxib or celecoxib [61,62]. Additionally, in a large randomized trial of individuals who had rheumatoid arthritis or osteoarthritis, study participants who took celecoxib had fewer symptomatic upper-GI ulcers and ulcer complications than individuals who took ibuprofen or diclofenac over the first 6 months of use, although this benefit disappeared by the end of a year of use [63,64]. This observation is particularly important, because few individuals who take NSAIDs regularly are expected to be on these drugs for less than a year.

Opioids

Opioids are the cornerstone of the analgesic regimen for moderate-to-severe pain, though not all individuals will respond similarly. As a result, close follow-up and regular assessment are necessary. Opioid is the preferred name for this class of analgesics, because narcotic is primarily a legal term used to refer to drugs from various pharmacologic classes and is associated with important psychological barriers to pain management [63]. Opioids and related drugs may be described in several ways, including their activity at opioid receptors, which is a proxy for potency. The three main types of opioid receptors that have been described so far are mu, delta, and kappa receptors [64,65]. Other receptors and subtypes are thought to exist also. The central and peripheral distribution of these receptors sometimes is used to suggest the function of compounds that interact preferentially with them, but this classification is relatively crude. Mu-receptor agonists generally produce analgesia, affect numerous body systems, and influence mood and reward behavior [64,65]. Delta-receptor agonists also act as analgesics, although none of the currently available opioids are mainly kappa-receptor active. Kappa-receptor agonists are also analgesics and may cause less respiratory depression and miosis; however, these compounds also have psychological effects and can produce dysphoria. In the dosage range typically used to treat patients who have acute postoperative pain, mu-receptor agonists have no therapeutic ceiling effect [64,65]. Therefore, unlike nonopioid analgesics, dosages of these drugs can be adjusted upward until satisfactory pain control is achieved or adverse effects become intolerable. Opioids lack the adverse GI, renal, and hematologic effects of NSAIDs, and the inability to attain sufficient analgesia with one opioid does not preclude the use of another.

Most of the commonly used opioids are mu-receptor agonists, although drugs may interact with more than one type of receptor, and receptors themselves may interact [64,65]. For example, several drugs are mu-receptor antagonists and kappa-receptor agonists. The mu-receptor antagonist–kappa-receptor agonist drugs were designed to cause less respiratory depression and to have a lower potential for abuse; however, at equianalgesic doses, the adverse effect profile of these drugs is similar to that of mu-receptor agonists [64,65]. The clinical implication is that although-receptor agonists typically have a linear dose–response relationship, mu-receptor antagonist–kappa-receptor agonist drugs are thought to have a ceiling effect, above which pain may increase because of mu-receptor antagonism. As a result, mu-receptor antagonist–kappa-receptor agonist opioids are not considered appropriate for first-line use for postoperative pain and generally are not considered appropriate for the treatment of persistent pain [14]. Box 1 lists opioid analgesics that are available in the United States.

Opioid pharmacokinetics

Although little attention generally is paid to the clinical pharmacokinetics of opioids, differences may matter, particularly those in time to onset of action and bioavailability, which sometimes are misinterpreted as differences in potency. Tables 1 and 2 summarize selected pharmacokinetic variables for intravenous and oral opioids, respectively.

The pharmacokinetic properties of an opioid can dictate the circumstances under which its use is most appropriate. Lipid-soluble drugs such as fentanyl, which diffuse rapidly across the blood–brain barrier, are preferable if analgesia is required immediately before a short, painful procedure. Differences in pharmacokinetics can be used to clinical advantage by changing the formulation or the route of administration. In addition, the elimination half-life of each opioid except methadone is short enough that steady state is reached in about a day or less. Thus, doses can be adjusted at least once a day with some confidence that the ultimate analgesic effect of the dose is being observed.

Equianalgesic dosage conversion

Although morphine is considered the standard of opioid analgesia, patients who do not respond to optimal doses or who have unmanageable adverse effects may respond well to an equianalgesic dosage of

---

Box 1. Opioid analgesics available in the United States, by receptor activity

Mu agonists
Alfentanil
Codeine
Hydrocodone
Hydromorphone
Fentanyl
Levorphanol
Meperidine
Methadone
Morphine
Opium
Oxycodone
Oxymorphone
Remifentanil
Sufentanil
Tramadol

Kappa agonist/mu antagonists
Butorphanol
Nalbuphine
Pentazocine

Mu antagonists
Nalmefene
Naloxone
Naltrexone

Mu partial agonist/kappa antagonist
Buprenorphine

---

hydromorphone, oxycodone, fentanyl, oxymorphone, or methadone. Similarly, an individual who has diminished renal function may benefit from drugs without clinically significant active metabolites, such as oxycodone or hydromorphone (or fentanyl, methadone).

At equianalgesic dosages, full opioid agonists have similar efficacy but may differ in their adverse effects. Equianalgesic dosage conversion tables commonly use an intramuscular dose of 10 mg morphine sulfate as the basis for comparing alternative routes and opioids, but conversions are approximate and generally are based on limited evidence from studies of acute pain in young, otherwise healthy individuals. Just as patients may vary in their response to a certain opioid, they also may require higher or lower conversion factors than those suggested, especially for opioid-tolerant patients.

Table 1
Selected clinical pharmacokinetic parameters of commonly used intravenous opioids

Drug	Approximate time to onset (min)	Approximate time to peak (min)	Approximate duration (h)	Dose equivalency (mg)[a]
Fentanyl	1–2	5	1–2	0.01
Hydromorphone	2–3	10–15	Approximately 2	0.2
Meperidine	10	30	3–4	10
Methadone	2–3	5–6	6–12	1
Morphine	2–4	15–20	Approximately 2	1
Oxymorphone	5–10	60–120	Approximately 3–6	0.3

[a] On a milligram-to-milligram basis relative to morphine, fentanyl is approximately 100 times more potent; hydromorphone is approximately five times more potent. Meperidine is approximately 1/10 as potent, and oxymorphone is approximately three times more potent.

Methadone is a good example of this phenomenon. Although methadone typically is considered to be equipotent to morphine in opioid-inexperienced persons, methadone dosages often need to be reduced dramatically over the first few days of use because of the drug's long elimination half-life and activity at the N-methyl D-aspartate receptor. Substantial decreases (approximately 90%) in the methadone dosage may be needed over the first few days after agents are switched. This property of methadone is critically important; overlooking it can contribute to serious or fatal adverse events.

There are various ways to achieve conversion to an alternative drug or route. Two such methods are shown in Tables 3 and 4, with examples in

Table 2
Selected clinical pharmacokinetic parameters of commonly used oral opioids

Drug name	Approximate time to onset (min)	Approximate time to peak (h)	Approximate duration (h)	Approximate bioavailability (%)
Hydromorphone	30–45	1.5–2	3–4	60
Meperidine	30–45	1.5	3	30
Methadone	30	2–3	6–12	80
Morphine sulfate (immediate-release, sublingual)	30–45	1.5–2	3–4	30
Morphine sulfate (long-acting)				
MS Contin, Oramorph SR	120	6–8	10–12	30
Kadian	120	8–12	18–24	30
Avinza	45	4–6	18–24	30
Oxycodone (immediate-release)	20–45	1.5–2	3–4	80
Oxycodone (controlled-release)	30–60	4–6	10–12	80
Oxymorphone (IR)	NA	NA	3–6	10
Oxymorphone (CR)	NA	1–2	~12	10

Table 3
Equianalgesic conversion chart

	Parenteral (mg)	Oral (mg)	Duration (h)
Codeine	120	200	3–4
Hydromorphone	1.5	7.5	2–4
Meperidine	75	300	2–4
Methadone[a]	5	10	6–8
Morphine	10	30	2–4
Oxycodone	NA	20	2–4

[a] Note that although methadone is approximately equipotent to morphine, it is substantially more bioavailable, has an extended elimination half-life, and has activity at the N-methyl D-aspartate receptor. As a result, methadone doses typically need to be significantly reduced (approximately 90%) within the first few days of treatment to avoid accumulation of drug and serious or fatal adverse effects.

Data from Ashburn MA, Lipman AG, Carr D, et al. Principles of analgesic use in the treatment of acute pain and chronic pain. 5th edition. Glenview (IL): American Pain Society; 2003.

Appendix 1. More comprehensive reviews of equianalgesic dosage conversion can be found elsewhere [67,68]. It is important to note that equianalgesic conversions are estimates that may vary substantially, depending on the method of calculation used. For example, conversion from intravenous morphine to oral oxycodone by using method 1 in Table 4 indicates that 48 mg of intravenous morphine sulfate is equivalent to 96 mg of oral oxycodone hydrochloride, while the approach described in method 2 in Table 4 provides a result of 60 mg of oral oxycodone hydrochloride. In addition, oral oxycodone hydrochloride 20 mg is considered equivalent to 30 mg of oral morphine sulfate. Although this method is used widely, for this conversion factor to be correct, oxycodone would have to be 50% rather than 80% bioavailable [36]. In clinical practice, various approaches often are used to help avoid overdoses while providing appropriate pain relief. These measures include adjusting dosages to account for incomplete cross-tolerance (often a 25% to 50% decrease in the dosage of the new drug) and using a portion of the calculated equianalgesic dosage on a scheduled basis, and allowing the patient to receive the remainder of the expected daily analgesic requirement as rescue doses on a liberal as-needed basis.

While the full mu-receptor agonist opioids provide similar analgesia in equipotent doses, three of these drugs are best avoided whenever possible: meperidine, propoxyphene, and codeine.

Meperidine

Meperidine has a low potency relative to morphine, a short duration of action, and a toxic metabolite, normeperidine. A common postoperative dose of meperidine hydrochloride is 75 mg, but this dose is equivalent to about 5 to 7.5 mg of morphine sulfate. Furthermore, the prescribed dose

Table 4
Equianalgesic dose conversion methods for opioids

Method 1 [66]	Method 2 [36]
1. Total the 24-hour dose of current drug, including all breakthrough doses.	1. Total the 24-hour dose that produces adequate analgesia.
2. Convert for drug and route by using an equianalgesic dosage conversion table.	2. Convert the 24-hour total dose to a morphine- equivalent dose by using a conversion factor of 1 for morphine, methadone, and oxycodone; 10 for meperidine, 0.2 for hydromorphone, and 0.01 for fentanyl. On a milligram-to-milligram basis, methadone, morphine, and oxycodone are approximately equipotent; meperidine is approximately 1/10 as potent as morphine. Hydromorphone is approximately five times as potent as morphine, and fentanyl is approximately 100 times as potent as morphine.
Because methadone has a long elimination half-life, is approximately 80% bioavailable, and is active at the N-methyl D-aspartate receptor, doses may need to be reduced substantially (approximately 90%) over the first few days after switching from another opioid.	Because methadone has a long elimination half-life, is approximately 80% bioavailable, and is active at the N-methyl D-aspartate receptor, doses may need to be reduced substantially (approximately 90%) over the first few days after switching from another opioid.
3. Divide the total 24-hour dose of the new drug by the schedule for the new drug.	3. Adjust the 24-hour dose of opioid for bioavailability. Methadone and oxycodone are approximately 80% bioavailable; hydromorphone is approximately 60% bioavailable, and meperidine and morphine are approximately 30% bioavailable.
4. For opioid-tolerant persons, consider reducing the calculated dose of the new drug by 25% to 50% to account for incomplete cross-tolerance.	4. Adjust the dose of the new drug based on its elimination half-life. From clinical experience, the approximate duration of effect for meperidine is 3 hours; for immediate-release hydromorphone, morphine and oxycodone, 3 to 4 hours; for methadone, 6–12 hours; for controlled-release morphine and oxycodone, 10 to 12 hours.
5. Calculate a dose for breakthrough pain: 10% to 20% of the total daily opioid dose, or 25% to 30% of a single regularly scheduled dose.	5. Calculate a dose for breakthrough pain: 10% to 20% of the total daily opioid dose, or 25% to 30% of a single regularly scheduled dose.

frequency is often every 4 to 6 hours, but meperidine produces pain relief for 2.5 to 3 hours, so, to provide pain relief equivalent to 10 mg of morphine sulfate every 4 hours, 100 to 150 mg of meperidine hydrochloride would be needed every 3 hours [66].

Normeperidine is the major metabolite of meperidine and is a neurotoxic compound that can cause dysphoria, nervousness, tremors, myoclonus, and generalized seizures [63,69–71]. Normeperidine is eliminated renally, which increases the risk of seizures in patients who have decreased renal function, such as the elderly; however, seizures also have been observed in patients who have normal renal function [66]. The half-life of normeperidine in patients who have normal renal function is 15 to 30 hours [66]. Normeperidine is half as potent as meperidine as an analgesic but is two to three times as potent as a convulsant [63,69]. Concomitant therapy with monoamine oxidase inhibitors, including selegiline and meperidine, or use of meperidine within 2 weeks of discontinuation of a monoamine oxidase inhibitor (MAOI), can result in serotonin syndrome, whose symptoms include hypertensive crisis, hyperpyrexia, and fatal cardiovascular system collapse [70].

For patients who experience neurotoxicities caused by meperidine and its metabolite, an antagonist such as naloxone should not be used, because naloxone does not reverse the effects of normeperidine and may increase seizure activity [63,69]. To treat seizures as a result of meperidine use, discontinuation of meperidine and substitution with an alternate mu-receptor agonist opioid is recommended, and an anticonvulsant like diazepam or phenytoin can be used to control seizures. Because of meperidine's numerous disadvantages, it should not be used as first-line therapy for postoperative pain management, and the American Pain Society (APS) now recommends avoiding meperidine for the treatment of acute or cancer pain whenever possible [66]. It should be avoided for persistent noncancer pain as well. Meperidine should be used only for short courses in patients who have had an allergic or intolerable reaction to other agents. When avoiding meperidine is not possible, APS recommends that it be used for no longer than 48 hours at dosages not greater than 600 mg intravenously in 24 hours in patients who have normal renal function [66]. Meperidine use also should be avoided in patients who have impaired renal function (creatinine clearance, less than 50 mL/min), pre-existing convulsive disorder, and known atrial flutter or supraventricular tachycardia [63,69].

Propoxyphene

Propoxyphene generally is used to treat mild-to-moderate pain, but because of toxicities associated with this drug and its primary metabolite, norpropoxyphene, its use should be limited [63,72]. Norpropoxyphene can cause severe adverse effects, such as cardiotoxicity and pulmonary edema. The half-life of propoxyphene is 6 to 12 hours, and that of norpropoxyphene is 30 to 36 hours; thus, drug concentrations and the potential for toxicity are increased in patients who have decreased renal function or are receiving repeated doses. Additionally, older persons are at increased risk of falls and related injuries because of the central nervous-system adverse effects [73]. Kamal-Bahl and colleagues [74] published the results of a cohort database study that included 363,503 patients with a mean follow-up of 464 days. They found that propoxyphene users had twofold higher risk for hip fracture ([hazard ratio] [95% CI]. 2.05 [1.87-2.25]) compared with nonusers of analgesics. Therefore, many institutions restrict the use of propoxyphene, particularly in patients older than 65 years of age. In addition, propoxyphene has no clinical advantage over nonopioid analgesics, such as acetaminophen [6,75]. Despite recommendations to avoid the use of propoxyphene in older adults, its use continues to occur in a higher proportion of patients aged 65 years or older than in younger patients [76].

Codeine

Codeine must be converted to morphine by means of the cytochrome P-450 2D6 pathway to provide analgesia [77]. A substantial percentage of Caucasians are poor metabolizers of this isoenzyme and are not able to convert codeine to morphine; these patients receive no benefit from codeine, although they are still at risk for adverse effects [65]. In addition, adverse effects such as nausea and constipation occur more frequently with codeine than with other agents at equianalgesic dosages [66].

Contraindications

Although genuine allergy to opioids is thought to be rare, the use of an opioid from the same chemical class as an opioid to which a patient has a documented allergy is contraindicated. Under these circumstances, an opioid from another class should be chosen. Most of the full mu-receptor agonists are phenanthrenes, while alfentanil, fentanyl, meperidine, remifentanil, and sufentanil are phenylpiperidines, and methadone and propoxyphene are diphenylpropylamines [65]. Patients may report having an opioid allergy when they have had an opioid-related adverse effect. A diagnosis of allergy can be compromised further by the fact that many opioids cause histamine release.

Adverse effects of opioids

Few data support differences in adverse effects among opioids at equianalgesic dosages for postoperative pain [67,77–79]. Study results are often difficult to interpret because of the use of nonequianalgesic dosages or by the fact that pain itself can cause adverse effects, including nausea. Differences in the rate of adverse effects may be a consequence of individual patient characteristics [80]. Opioid metabolites also may cause adverse effects [78,79]. For example, morphine-6-glucuronide, the primary active metabolite of morphine, may accumulate in patients who have diminished renal function and can contribute to analgesia, and adverse effects, including cognitive impairment, myoclonus, and hyperalgesia. Adverse effects attributed to the meperidine metabolite normeperidine also are documented, including dysphoria, excitation, and seizures, especially in the elderly or patients who have renal dysfunction, even with short-term administration [66,69,70,81].

Although active metabolites of other opioids have been discovered, there is less evidence to support their implication in adverse effects similar to those seen with normeperidine.

The adverse effects most commonly associated with opioids are respiratory depression, sedation, nausea, vomiting, constipation, urinary retention, and itching [65,82]. Other adverse effects include confusion, hallucinations, nightmares, multifocal myoclonus, and dizziness. Factors such as age, extent of disease, concurrent administration of certain drugs, prior opioid administration, and route of administration also can increase the risk of opioid-related adverse effects.

Respiratory depression

Respiratory depression is the most serious adverse effect of opioids, which cause this effect by acting directly on respiratory centers [65]. Therapeutic dosages of morphine can affect respiratory rate, minute volume, and tidal exchange. As carbon dioxide (CO_2) accumulates, it stimulates central chemoreceptors, resulting in a compensatory increase in the respiratory rate. Opioids, however, shift the CO_2 response curve so that the level of CO_2 needed to stimulate respiration becomes higher. Equianalgesic dosages of other opioids produce the same degree of respiratory depression, and the effect increases with the dosage. Patients who have impaired respiratory function, sleep apnea, or bronchial asthma are at increased risk for respiratory depression. Therefore, these individuals should be monitored carefully. Opioid-induced respiratory depression sometimes is defined clinically as a function of respiratory rate or the partial pressure of arterial carbon dioxide ($paCO_2$), but these measures by themselves are not very specific indicators of respiratory depression [63]. In addition, the rate of change in respiratory rate or $paCO_2$ may be more important than the absolute rate or concentration. To get around this issue, some clinicians advocate monitoring for sedation. Table 5 shows an example of a sedation scale.

Table 5
Sedation scale

Sedation score	How sleepy or drowsy?	How arousable?
0	Not	Easy
1	Occasional or infrequent	Easy
2	Frequent	Easy
3	Frequent	Not easy
S	Normal sleep	Normal sleep

A sedation score of 2 is similar to normal sleep, but implies an opioid-induced process.
Data from Pasero C, Portenoy RK, McCaffery M. Opioid analgesics. In: McCaffery M, Pasero C, editors. Pain: clinical manual. 2nd edition. St. Louis (MO): Mosby; 1999. p. 161–299.

When respiratory depression does occur, it is often in opioid-inexperienced patients who have received a brief course of an opioid and have other signs, such as sedation and mental clouding [63,72]. Respiratory depression generally occurs more rapidly with lipid-soluble agents, and with large rapid dose escalation. Although tolerance to this effect generally occurs with repeated use of opioids, measuring the respiratory rate and monitoring for signs of respiratory depression in patients receiving opioids are recommended, especially in patients who have not received opioids previously. Additionally, if naloxone is used, its dosage should be adjusted slowly to reverse respiratory depression and decrease the chance of antagonizing analgesic effects. One way to achieve this is to dilute 0.4 mg (1 mL) of naloxone hydrochloride to a volume of 10 mL, and then give the patient 1 mL (40 µg) of this solution at a time. Adverse effects related to naloxone include:

The individual's pain may recur (after the naloxone concentration falls).
If a large bolus dose of naloxone is given, severe worsening pain may occur that may be difficult to treat.
Opioid withdrawal may occur in patients who have opioid physical dependence.
Hypertension, tachycardia, and pulmonary edema may result. as well as seizures if naloxone is administered after receiving meperidine [63,69].

Furthermore, if naloxone is given to reverse opioid-induced respiratory depression from a long-acting opioid, care must be taken to monitor the patient, because naloxone is relatively short-acting, and to avoid a recurrence of opioid-induced respiratory depression. An intravenous naloxone drip may be needed.

Nausea and vomiting

Nausea and vomiting are the most common and, from the patient's perspective, least desirable postoperative adverse effects of opioids [83]. Postoperative opioid use can contribute to these adverse effects by directly stimulating the chemoreceptor trigger zone, depressing the vomiting center, and slowing GI motility [65,84]. The frequency of nausea and vomiting is higher in ambulatory patients, suggesting that this effect has a vestibular component. Antiemetics, such as transdermal scopolamine, metoclopramide, or droperidol, can be used along with the opioid, and in severe cases, a serotonin type 3-receptor antagonist may be useful [84]. The use of phenothiazines as antiemetics is common, but they often cause sedation.

Constipation

Opioids cause constipation by acting on multiple sites in the GI tract and spinal cord to produce a decrease in peristalsis and intestinal secretions, resulting in dry stools and constipation. This in turn may result in decreased willingness to take analgesics [65]. Tolerance to this effect generally develops slowly, if at all. As a result, patients taking an opioid also should be given prophylactic laxatives. Although bowel regimens consisting of only a stool softener (ie, docusate sodium) are used commonly, this practice should be discouraged, because opioids slow normal peristalsis. Using only a stool softener is expected to result in an uncomfortable patient who is unable to evacuate his or her bowels. Instead, a bowel regimen consisting of a stool softener and a stimulant laxative, such as senna, is preferred.

Urinary retention

Opioids may possess actions that can affect the bladder, including increased smooth muscle tone (with potential bladder spasms) and increased sphincter tone, (which may lead to resulting in urinary retention) [65]. This adverse event generally occurs more frequently in older adults, and can require catheterization to manage. As a result, prevention and assessment are important.

Itching

The mechanism by which opioids cause itching is not fully known, although the release of histamine from mast cells is thought to contribute [84]. Histamine release explains only part of the problem, however, because itching still occurs with opioids that do not cause histamine release, like fentanyl. Opioids also may cause itching through their ability to disinhibit itch-specific neurons. To relieve itching, switching to a different opioid may be effective. Itching by itself does not necessarily require that an opioid from a different chemical class be chosen; however, if the itching is accompanied by a rash, allergy cannot be ruled out. In such a case, an opioid from a different chemical class is recommended. An antihistamine, such as diphenhydramine, may be useful, although less sedating agents, such as hydroxyzine or cyproheptadine, may be preferable [84]. Nalbuphine also can be of value, but it has the potential to lead to other opioid-related adverse effects, and theoretically may increase pain through mu-receptor antagonism.

Summary

The promise of relief from suffering exerts a powerful attraction, calling people in distress to seek medical care. Pain is a universal part of being human, and yet, there is ample evidence that many people from all backgrounds, stages of life, and levels of health care experience receive less than optimal treatment of their pain. Pharmacotherapy is an important part of its treatment, and through better understanding of how these tools are used, there are important opportunities to help reduce suffering of individuals with pain.

Appendix 1

Equianalgesic conversion examples [36,66,67]

1. A patient is receiving intravenous morphine 2 mg/h continuous infusion and has received six breakthrough doses of 1 mg within the last 24 hours. The patient is now able to tolerate oral medication. Convert the patient's opioid regimen to oral controlled-release oxycodone using data in Table 3.

   Step 1—Total the 24 hour dose of current drug, including all breakthrough doses: 2 mg × 24 hours = 48 mg. Six breakthrough doses × 1 mg = 6 mg. Total daily dose = 54 mg

   Step 2—Convert 24 hour dose to new drug and/or route using an equianalgesic conversion table: 10 mg intravenous morphine = 20 mg oral oxycodone Multiply 54 mg × conversion factor of 2 (20/10) Total 24 hour dose of oxycodone = 108 mg

   Step 3—Divide the total dose of new drug by the schedule of the new drug: Controlled-release oxycodone is usually dosed every 12 hours. 108/2 = 54 mg every 12 hours Closest dose available is 40 mg tablet + 10 mg tablet = 50 mg

   Step 4—In opioid-tolerant patients, consider reducing calculated dose of the new drug by 33% to 50% to account for incomplete cross-tolerance: If situation warrants, reduce 54 mg by 33% to 50% = 27–36 mg. May choose 20 mg tablet + 10 mg tablet = 30 mg

   Step 5—Calculate a breakthrough dose: either 10% to 20% of the total daily opioid dose or 25% to 30% of the single-standing dose: If one chooses the 50 mg dose, and decides to administer 20% of total daily dose, breakthrough dose = 20 mg. Immediate-release oxycodone usually is scheduled every 6 hours, but can be given more frequently.

   New regimen

   Oxycodone controlled-release tablets 50 mg every 12 hours, plus oxycodone immediate-release tablets 20 mg every 6 hours as required for breakthrough pain

2. A patient is comfortable receiving an intravenous infusion of morphine 2 mg per hour. How should a prescription for oral oxycodone be ordered?

   Morphine 2 mg/hr intravenously = 48 mg/24 hours

   48 mg intravenous morphine = 60 mg oral oxycodone (48/0.8)

   Prescribe: 5 mg oral oxycodone every 2 hours or 7.5 mg every 3 hours

3. A 24-hour dose of 18 mg of patient-controlled analgesia hydromorphone was needed for comfort. What dose of oral methadone is needed to maintain this effect?*

   18 mg intravenous hydromorphone × 5 = 90 mg intravenous morphine

   90 mg intravenous morphine = 90 mg intravenous methadone = 112.5 mg oral methadone (90/0.8)

   Approximately 25 mg every 6 hours or 35 mg every 8 hours

---

* Substantial decreases in dosing (approximately 90%) over the first few days of treatment generally are needed when converting to methadone.

References

[1] Middleton KR, Hing E. National Hospital Ambulatory Medical Care Survey: 2003 outpatient department summary. Advance data from vital and health statistics: no 366. Hyattsville (MD): National Center for Health Statistics; 2005.

[2] Gureje O, Von Korff M, Simon GE, et al. Persistent pain and well-being. A World Health Organization Study in primary care. JAMA 1998;280:147–51.

[3] Breivik H, Collett B, Ventafridda V, et al. Survey of chronic pain in Europe: prevalence, impact on daily life, and treatment. Eur J Pain 2006;10:287–333.

[4] Inpatient procedures. Fast stats A to Z. Available at: http://www.cdc.gov/nchs/fastats/insurg.htm. Accessed August 6, 2007.

[5] Cleeland CS, Gonin R, Hatfield AK, et al. Pain and its treatment in outpatients with metastatic cancer. N Engl J Med 1994;330:592–6.

[6] Carr DB, Jacox AK, Chapman CR, et al. Clinical practice guideline number 1: acute pain management: operative or medical procedures and trauma. Rockville (MD): Agency for Health Care Policy and Research; 1992, AHCPR publication no. 92-0032.

[7] Marks RM, Sachar EJ. Undertreatment of medical inpatients with narcotic analgesics. Ann Intern Med 1973;78:173–81.

[8] Donovan M, Dillon P, McGuire L. Incidence and characteristics of pain in a sample of medical–surgical inpatients. Pain 1987;30:69–78.

[9] Sriwatanakul K, Weis OF, Alloza JL, et al. Analysis of narcotic analgesic usage in the treatment of postoperative pain. JAMA 1983;250:926–9.

[10] Warfield CA, Kahn CH. Acute pain management: programs in US hospitals and experiences and attitudes among US adults. Anesthesiology 1995;83:1090–4.

[11] Miaskowski C, Nichols R, Brody R, et al. Assessment of patient satisfaction utilizing the American Pain Society's quality assurance standards on acute and cancer-related pain. J Pain Symptom Manage 1994;9:5–11.

[12] SUPPORT Principal Investigators. A controlled trial to improve care for seriously ill hospitalized patients. The study to understand prognoses and preferences for outcomes and risks of treatments (SUPPORT). JAMA 1995;274:1591–8.

[13] Wolfe J, Grier HE, Klar N, et al. Symptoms and suffering at the end of life in children with cancer. N Engl J Med 2000;342:326–33.

[14] Whelan CT, Jin L, Meltzer D. Pain and satisfaction with pain control in hospitalized medical patients. No such thing as low risk. Arch Intern Med 2004;164:175–80.

[15] Kehlet H. Surgical stress: the role of pain and analgesia. Br J Anaesth 1989;63:189–95.

[16] Gottschalk A, Smith DS, Jobes DR, et al. Preemptive epidural analgesia and recovery from radical prostatectomy. A randomized controlled trial. JAMA 1998;279:1076–82.

[17] Kiecolt-Glaser JK, Page GG, Marucha PT, et al. Psychological influences on surgical recovery: perspectives from psychoneuroimmunology. Am Psychol 1998;53:1209–18.

[18] Coley KC, Williams BA, DaPos SV, et al. Retrospective evaluation of unanticipated admissions and readmissions after same day surgery and associated costs. J Clin Anesth 2002;14:349–53.

[19] Cepeda MS, Africano JM, Polo R, et al. What decline in pain intensity is meaningful to patients with acute pain? Pain 2003;105(1–2):151–7.

[20] Bonica JJ. Importance of effective pain control. Acta Anaesthesiol Scand 1987;31(Suppl 85):1–16.

[21] Carr DB, Goudas L. Acute pain. Lancet 1999;353:2051–8.

[22] Kehlet H, Holte K. Effect of postoperative analgesia on surgical outcome. Br J Anaesth 2001;87:62–72.

[23] Strassels SA, Chen C, Carr DB. Postoperative analgesia: economics, resource use, and patient satisfaction in an urban teaching hospital. Anesth Analg 2002;94:130–7.

[24] Perkins FM, Kehlet H. Chronic pain as an outcome of surgery—a review of predictive factors. Anesthesiology 2000;93:1123–33.

[25] Stewart WF, Ricci JA, Chee E, et al. Lost productive time and cost due to common pain conditions in the US workforce. JAMA 2003;290:2443–54.

[26] Berger A, Dukes EM, Oster G. Clinical characteristics and economic costs of patients with painful neuropathic disorders. J Pain 2004;5:143–9.

[27] American Diabetes Association. Economic costs of diabetes in the US in 2002. Diabetes Care 2003;26:917–32.

[28] Gordois A, Scuffham P, Shearer A, et al. The health care costs of diabetic peripheral neuropathy in the US. Diabetes Care 2003;26:1790–5.

[29] Sleed M, Eccleston C, Beecham J, et al. The economic impact of chronic pain in adolescence: methodological considerations and a preliminary cost-of-illness study. Pain 2005;119: 183–90.

[30] Morris DB. The culture of pain. Berkeley (CA): University of California Press; 1993.

[31] Donabedian A. Evaluating the quality of medical care. Milbank Mem Fund Q 1966; 44(Suppl):166–206.

[32] Lasch K, Greenhill A, Wilkes G, et al. Why study pain? A qualitative analysis of medical and nursing faculty and students' knowledge of and attitudes to cancer pain management. J Palliat Med 2002;5:57–71.

[33] McNicol E. Pharmacy and pain management: much work left to do. J Am Pharm Assoc 2003;4343–4 [letter].

[34] Pain. International Association for the Study of Pain. IASP pain terminology. Available at: www.iasp-pain.org. Accessed August 6, 2007.

[35] Pasero C, Paice JA, McCaffery M. Basic mechanisms underlying the causes and effects of pain. In: McCaffery M, Pasero C, editors. Pain: clinical manual. 2nd edition. St. Louis (MO): Mosby; 1999. p. 15–34.

[36] Ready LB, Edwards WT, editors. Management of acute pain: a practical guide. Seattle (WA): IASP; 1992.

[37] Savage SR, Joranson DE, Covington EC, et al. Definitions related to the medical use of opioids: evolution towards universal agreement. J Pain Symptom Manage 2003;26: 655–67.

[38] McMahon SB, Koltzenburg M, editors. Wall & Melzack's textbook of pain. 5th edition. London: Elsevier Churchill Livingstone; 2006.

[39] McCaffery M. Pain control. Barriers to the use of available information. World Health Organization Expert Committee on Cancer Pain Relief and Active Supportive Care. Cancer 1992;70(Suppl 5):1438–49.

[40] Drayer RA, Henderson J, Reidenberg M. Barriers to better pain control in hospitalized patients. J Pain Symptom Manage 1999;17:434–40.

[41] Porter J, Jick H. Addiction rare in patients treated with narcotics. N Engl J Med 1980;302: 123.

[42] Perry S, Heidrich G. Management of pain during debridement: a survey of US burn units. Pain 1982;13:267–80.

[43] Brozovic M, Davies SC, Yardumian A, et al. Pain relief in sickle cell crisis. Lancet 1986;2: 624–5.

[44] Vichinsky EP, Johnson R, Lubin BH. Multidisciplinary approach to pain management in sickle cell disease. Am J Pediatr Hematol Oncol 1982;4:328–33.

[45] Pegelow CH. Survey of pain management therapy provided for children with sickle cell disease. Clin Pediatr 1992;31:211–4.

[46] Passik SD, Kirsh KL. The need to identify predictors of aberrant drug-related behavior and addiction in patients being treated with opioids for pain. Pain Med 2003;4: 186–9.

[47] Ballantyne JC, LaForge KS. Opioid dependence and addiction during opioid treatment of chronic pain. Pain 2007;129:235–55.

[48] Weissman DE, Haddox JD. Opioid pseudoaddiction—an iatrogenic syndrome. Pain 1989; 36:363–6.

[49] Bauer LA. Clinical pharmacokinetics and pharmacodynamics. In: DiPiro JT, Talbert RL, Yee GC, et al, editors. Pharmacotherapy: a pathophysiologic approach. New York: McGraw-Hill; 2005. p. 51–73.

[50] Lindblad CI, Gray SL, Guay DRP, et al. Geriatrics. In: DiPiro JT, Talbert RL, Yee GC, et al, editors. Pharmacotherapy: a pathophysiologic approach. New York: McGraw-Hill; 2005. p. 103–13.

[51] Hammerlein A, Derendorf H, Lowenthal DT. Pharmacokinetic and pharmacodynamic changes in the elderly: clinical implications. Clin Pharmacokinet 1998;35:49–64.

[52] Sotaniemi EA, Arranto AJ, Pelkonen O, et al. Age and cytochrome P-450-linked drug metabolism in humans. Clin Pharmacol Ther 1997;61:331–9.

[53] WHO's pain relief ladder. Available at: http://www.who.int/cancer/palliative/painladder/en/. Accessed August 6, 2007.

[54] Salicylates. Facts & comparisons 4.0. Available at: http://online.factsandcomparisons.com. Accessed August 5, 2007.

[55] Acetaminophen. Facts & comparisons 4.0. Available at: http://online.factsandcomparisons.com. Accessed August 5, 2007.

[56] Draganov P, Durrence H, Cox C, et al. Alcohol–acetaminophen syndrome. Postgrad Med 2000;107:189–95.

[57] Buck ML. Perioperative use of high-dose rectal acetaminophen. Pediatric Pharmacotherapy 2001;7:1–3.

[58] Birmingham PK, Tobin MJ, Henthorn TK, et al. Twenty-four-hour pharmacokinetics of rectal acetaminophen in children: an old drug with new recommendations. Anesthesiology 1997;87:244–52.

[59] Nonsteroidal anti-inflammatory drugs. Facts & comparisons 4.0. Available at: http://online.factsandcomparisons.com. Accessed August 5, 2007.

[60] Moote C. Efficacy of nonsteroidal anti-inflammatory drugs in the management of postoperative pain. Drugs 1992;44:14–30.

[61] Celebrex package insert. Available at: http://www.celebrex.com/pdf/Celebrex_PI.pdf. Accessed August 4, 2007.

[62] Schaefer MG, Plowman BK, Morreale AP, et al. Interaction of rofecoxib and celecoxib with warfarin. Am J Health Syst Pharm 2003;60:1319–23.

[63] Pasero C, Portenoy RK, McCaffery M. Opioid analgesics. In: McCaffery M, Pasero C, editors. Pain: clinical manual. 2nd edition. St. Louis (MO): Mosby; 1999. p. 161–299.

[64] Twycross RG. Opioids. In: Wall PD, Melzack R, editors. Textbook of pain. 4th edition. New York: Churchill Livingstone; 1999. p. 1187–214.

[65] Gutstein HB, Akil H. Opioid analgesics. In: Hardman JG, Limbird LE, Gilman AG, editors. Goodman and Gilman's the pharmacological basis of therapeutics. 10th edition. New York: McGraw-Hill; 2001. p. 569–619.

[66] Ashburn MA, Lipman AG, Carr D, et al. Principles of analgesic use in the treatment of acute pain and chronic pain. 5th edition. Glenview (IL): American Pain Society; 2003.

[67] Gammaitoni AR, Fine P, Alvarez N, et al. Clinical application of opioid equianalgesic data. Clin J Pain 2003;19:286–97.

[68] Souter KJ, Fitzgibbon D. Equianalgesic dose guidelines for long-term opioid use: theoretical and practical considerations. Seminars in anesthesia, perioperative medicine, and pain 2004; 23:271–80.

[69] Latta KS, Ginsberg B, Barkin RL. Meperidine: a critical review. Am J Ther 2002;9:53–68.

[70] Sporer K. The serotonin syndrome: implicated drugs, pathophysiology, and management. Drug Saf 1995;13:94–104.

[71] Michalets EL. Update: clinically significant cytochrome P-450 drug interactions. Pharmacotherapy 1998;18(1):84–112.

[72] Inturrisi CE. Clinical pharmacology of opioids for pain. Clin J Pain 2002;18:S3–13.

[73] Kamal-Bahal SJ, Doshi JA, Stuart BC, et al. Propoxyphene use by community dwelling and institutionalized elderly medicare beneficiaries. J Am Geriatr Soc 2003;51:1099–106.

[74] Kamal-Bahl SJ, Stuar BC, Beers MH. Propoxyphene use and risk for hip fractures in older adults. Am J Geriatr Pharmacother 2006;4:219–26.

[75] McQuay H, Moore A. Dextropropoxyphene in postoperative pain. In: McQuay H, Moore A, editors. An evidence-based resource in pain relief. New York: Oxford University Press; 1998. p. 132–7.

[76] Singh S, Sleeper RB, Seifert CF. Propoxyphene prescribing among populations older and younger than age 65 in a tertiary care hospital. Consult Pharm 2007;22:141–8.

[77] McQuay H. Opioids in pain management. Lancet 1999;353:2229–32.

[78] Sjogren P, Thunedborg LP, Christrup L, et al. Is development of hyperalgesia, allodynia, and myoclonus related to morphine metabolism during long-term administration? Six case histories. Acta Anaesthesiol Scand 1998;42:1070–5.

[79] Tiseo PJ, Thaler HT, Lapin J, et al. Morphine-6-glucuronide concentrations and opioid-related side effects: a survey in cancer patients. Pain 1995;61:47–54.

[80] Kalso E, Vainio A. Morphine and oxycodone hydrochloride in the management of cancer pain. Clin Pharmacol Ther 1990;47:639–46.

[81] Kaiko RF, Foley KM, Grabinski PY, et al. Central nervous system excitatory effects of meperidine in cancer patients. Ann Neurol 1983;13:180–5.

[82] Jacox A, Carr DB, Payne R, et al. Management of cancer pain: clinical practice guideline no. 9. Rockville (MD): Agency for Health Care Policy and Research; 1994, AHCPR publication no. 94-0592.

[83] Macario A, Weinger M, Carney S, et al. Which clinical anesthesia outcomes are important to avoid? The perspective of patients. Anesth Analg 1999;89:652–8.

[84] McNicol E, Horowicz-Mehler N, Fisk RA, et al. Management of opioid side effects in cancer-related and chronic noncancer pain: a systemic review. J Pain 2003;4:231–56.

ELSEVIER
SAUNDERS

CLINICS IN
GERIATRIC
MEDICINE

Clin Geriatr Med 24 (2008) 299–312

Topical Analgesic Agents

Gary McCleane, MD

Rampark Pain Centre, 2 Rampark, Lurgan, BT66 7JH, Northern Ireland, UK

Even to those who have an intimate and current knowledge of the mechanisms and transmission of pain generation, fully appreciating the complexities involved in these processes in different clinical scenarios can be daunting. Increased understanding of these mechanisms hopefully is matched by release of new pharmacologic agents that offer hope of pain relief for a greater number of patients, although, in reality, rapid advances in knowledge are accompanied by a more gradual release of new drugs. Not only do new drugs offer fresh hope but also novel formulations of old drugs can offer benefit and the realization that old drugs, originally developed for entirely different indications, can have useful pain-relieving effects.

There is a tendency in medicine that as the science that underpins practice becomes more detailed, more complex and invasive treatments are sought. This can offer benefit, but improving knowledge can highlight options for simpler, rather than more complex, treatments. This is demonstrated in the case of analgesics that achieve pain relief when applied topically. Increased knowledge now provides a scientific rationale as to why the topical application of certain agents provides pain relief and highlights other classes of drugs that have potential for having a topical analgesic effect.

The intention of this article is not to rehearse to readers the reasons why well-known topical analgesics are used, rather to highlight recent information about them and, more importantly, suggest a range of other drugs that have a topical mode of action and indicate how they can be used clinically. With some of these more novel options, a considerable body of animal and human data underpins their use. For others, the suggestions are based on more speculative evidence.

Perhaps the fundamental question that needs to be asked is why the topical route of administration must be considered at all. Two major reasons exist. First, if the intention of therapy is to maximize drug concentration

E-mail address: gary@mccleane.freeserve.co.uk

at particular target tissues (nerve fibers, receptors, and so forth) in order to maximize therapeutic effect yet minimize drug concentrations at other more distant areas (hence, minimize the risk for side effects), and if these target tissues have a high peripheral concentration and are localized, then topical administration seems an attractive proposition. Second, patients like the concept of applying medication to where they are sore.

The difference between topical and transdermal administration of drugs is highlighted. Topical implies the application of a drug to a painful area and that the effect of the drug is local rather than systemic. Transdermal implies the application of the drug to the skin as a way of achieving a systemic concentration and, hence, systemic effect from that drug.

In the context of pain management in elderly patients, the issue of side effects of drugs and the propensity of these drugs to interact with other concomitant medication becomes particularly important. It often is easy to suggest analgesic options for pain relief in elderly patients but more difficult to find drugs that do not impose intolerable side effects on these patients or have deleterious effects on drugs taken for other conditions. Several topical analgesic options have the possibility of providing pain relief and doing away with the need to consider more toxic oral alternatives.

Individual classes of drugs and how they may have a role in pain management when applied topically are discussed.

Nonsteroidal anti-inflammatory drugs

Topical nonsteroidal anti-inflammatory drugs (NSAIDs) are effective and safe in the management of acute pain [1]. That does not mean that they help all patients. Mason and colleagues [1] found that on analysis of 26 trials, including 2853 patients who had acute pain, the number needed to treat was 3.8. Therefore, if pain relief is not apparent, sustained use of topical NSAIDs is not justifiable.

One impediment to the use of topical NSAIDs is that, to date, most preparations are immediate release and tend to be gels; therefore, administration of a measured dose is difficult because of the application of varying quantities of the gel and because it is rubbed off the application area easily before absorption occurs. Several patch formulations are under examination, including patches containing ketoprofen [2], naproxen [3], and diclofenac [4], and alternative gel formulations, such as the use of lecithin organogel with aceclofenac [5]. These may allow a more measured application of drug.

Perhaps one of the major problems with topical NSAID use is the danger of polypharmacy, particularly as so many NSAIDs are sold over the counter in topical and oral forms. Topical NSAIDs produce high dermal concentrations of an NSAID, whereas adjacent muscle levels are as high when an NSAID is given systemically [6]. Gastrointestinal side effects occur less frequently than when a drug is given orally but are more likely in patients who previously had such side effects in response to oral NSAIDs [7].

Local anesthetics

Skin infiltration with local anesthetic is a tried and tested method of providing skin anesthesia and analgesia. It is impractical, however, for long-term use. Several local anesthetic preparations now are available that are applied topically. Amethocaine is presented as a gel, whereas a mixture of local anesthetics (lidocaine and prilocaine) is available in cream form and is used widely to provide skin anesthesia before venipuncture. It also can be of value in reducing the pain associated with other procedures, such as lumbar puncture, intramuscular injection, and even circumcision [8]. Although the eutectic mixture of local anesthetics does not have United States Food and Drug Administration approval for any neuropathic pain condition, several uncontrolled studies suggest it can reduce the pain of postherpetic neuralgia [9,10], although another randomized, controlled study of the same condition fails to show any benefit [11].

Lidocaine also is available in a 5% patch formulation that has approval for use in postherpetic neuralgia [12,13]. It also may reduce pain from a wide variety of other sources, including painful polyneuropathy [14] and osteoarthritis [15]. The amount of lidocaine actually absorbed is small and well below that which leads to systemic side effects. The safety margin is so great that several patches can be used simultaneously with no loss of safety.

Capsaicin

Capsaicin has the potential of reducing pain by reversibly depleting sensory nerve endings of substance P [16,17] and by reversibly reducing the density of epidermal nerve fibers [18]. It is available commercially as a 0.025% and a 0.075% cream. It reduces the pain of diabetic neuropathy [19–22], postherpetic neuralgia [23–25], surgical neuropathic pain [26], chronic distal painful polyneuropathy [27], osteoarthritis [28–33], and neck pain [34].

In practice, repeated application of capsaicin is required before clinical effect may be apparent. The major side effect associated with use is a burning, tingling sensation and allodynia at the application site. Although usually this settles with repeated use, it can be of a severity that significantly reduces compliance. Other side effects include sneezing, which seems to be associated with excessive use, drying of the cream, and aerosolization of the dried cream irritating the nasal mucosa. Accidental application to other areas of the body also can cause discomfort.

Several strategies can be used to reduce the burning discomfort of application. These include preadministration of ketamine [35] or lidocaine 5%

cream [36] or the coadministration of glyceryl trinitrate (GTN) [32,37,38], which also can enhance the analgesic effect of the capsaicin [32].

Nitrates

Traditionally, nitrates have been used in the management of angina pectoris. Among the preparations available are GTN ointment and transdermal patches. In addition to this conventional use, topical nitrates are useful topical analgesics. Although the ointment form is messy to apply and easy to overuse, hence precipitating a nitrate headache, the patch formulations allow a more precisely measured dose to be used. Among the potential benefits of their use are their safety and the fact that they can allow avoidance of NSAIDs with all their potential for adverse effects, particularly in elderly subjects.

Exogenous nitrates stimulate the release of nitric oxide (NO) [39]. This substance is a potent mediator in a variety of different cellular systems, such as the endothelium and the central and peripheral nervous system. It is released from the endothelium and from neutrophils and macrophages, all involved intimately in the inflammatory process. It seems that NO exerts its effect by stimulating increases in guanylate cyclase, thereby increasing levels of 3',5',cyclic GMP [40]. Cholinergic drugs, such as acetylcholine, produce analgesia in a similar fashion by releasing NO and increasing NO at the nociceptor level [41]. In addition to these actions, NO may activate ATP-sensitive potassium channels and activate peripheral antinociception [42].

From a clinical perspective, topical GTN can reduce the pain from any inflammatory condition that is superficial and localized. Therefore, it reduces pain from chronic supraspinatus tendonitis [43,44], osteoarthritis [32,45], and infusion-related thrombophlebitis [46]. It also can reduce the pain and inflammation associated with the sclerotherapy of varicose veins [47] and has an analgesic effect in patients who have vulvar pain [48].

It is contended, therefore, that topical nitrates should have an important role in the management of localized pain in elderly patients, particularly as they may reduce reliance on other potentially more toxic analgesic classes.

Tricyclic antidepressants

It is established firmly that oral tricyclic antidepressant (TCA) drugs can relieve a variety of types of pain, in particular those that are neuropathic. Unfortunately, they also have a substantial risk for causing side effects and, therefore, their suitability for use in elderly patients is at times questionable. Tricyclics can relieve pain by a variety of actions. Most well known are their effects of augmenting descending noradrenergic and serotinergic inhibitory drives. They also have effects on central opioid and N-methyl-D-aspartate (NMDA) receptors. None of these explains the observation that small quantities of TCAs can relieve pain when applied topically. It seems, however, that TCAs also have other effects.

At peripheral nerve terminals in rodents, adenosine A_1 receptor activation produces antinociception by decreasing cyclic AMP levels in the sensory nerve terminals, whereas adenosine A_2 receptor activation produces pronociception by increasing cyclic AMP levels in the sensory nerve terminals. Adenosine A_3 receptor activation produces pain behaviors resulting from the release of histamine and serotonin from mast cells and subsequent actions in the sensory nerve terminals [49]. Caffeine acts as a nonspecific adenosine receptor antagonist. When systemic caffeine is administered with systemic amitriptyline, the normal effect on thermal hyperalgesia is blocked. When amitriptyline is administered into a rodent paw that has neuropathic pain, an antihyperalgesic effect is recorded (but not when given into the contralateral paw). This antihyperalgesic effect is blocked by caffeine [50], suggesting that at least part of the effect of peripherally applied amitriptyline is mediated through peripheral adenosine receptors.

This is not the only peripheral action of TCAs. When a TCA is injected into a rat sciatic notch, complete sciatic nerve block ensues. When compared with the local anesthetic, bupivicaine, the TCAs, amitriptyline, doxepin, and imipramine, produce a longer complete sciatic nerve block, although the block produced by trimipramine and desipramine is shorter than that produced by bupivicaine [51]. When amitriptyline is applied topically, it produces longer cutaneous analgesia than lidocaine [52]. These findings suggest that TCAs also posses sodium channel-blocking effects.

When TCAs are applied topically in animal pain models, confirmation of an antinociceptive effect is observed. Using the classic chronic nerve constriction model for neuropathic pain, topically applied amitriptyline has an antinociceptive effect when applied to the paw ipsilateral to the side of injury. When applied to the contralateral paw, no antinociception is measurable [53,54], suggesting a local, rather than systemic, antinociceptive effect. Similar results are observed when desipramine is used but not when fluoxetine is examined [55].

Another animal pain model is the formalin model of chronic inflammation. When formalin is applied to a rodent paw, a biphasic response is observable and measurable. When amitriptyline [56–58] or desipramine [55] is coapplied with the formalin, the magnitude of both phases is reduced. When amitriptyline is administered peripherally along with formalin, Fos immunoreactivity in the dorsal region of the spinal cord is significantly lower than in animals in which formalin is administered alone [58].

Su and Gebhart [59] showed that when induced visceral pain is considered, peripherally administered imipramine, desipramine, and clomipramine reduced the response to noxious colorectal distension by 20%, 22%, and 46%, respectively, when compared with control-treated animals.

One last animal model to consider is that of induced thermal injury to the paw. When amitriptyline is applied to a rodent paw at the time of thermal

injury, antihyperalgesic and analgesic effects are observed. When amitriptyline is applied after injury, analgesic, but not antihyperalgesic, effects are
observed [60]. These animal findings are consistent with human observation
and study. Several randomized trials in human subjects who had neuropathic
pain show statistically significant reductions in pain scores when topical 5%
doxepin was applied. Maximum effect was observed after 2 weeks' treatment
and side effects were infrequent and mild. In particular, those side effects
associated with oral use of TCAs were observed infrequently [61,62]. Case
report evidence also suggests that topically applied 5% doxepin cream can
reduce the symptoms of complex regional pain syndrome type 1 [63], and
when doxepin is used as an oral rinse in patients who have oral pain as a result
of cancer or cancer treatment, useful pain reduction is observed [64].

It is suggested, therefore, that topical application of a TCA may be
a treatment method for patients who have localized pain, whereas in other
circumstances, an oral TCA may be considered. Repeated application of
small volumes of cream are required but when used in this fashion, a local
effect can be obtained and systemic side effects noted commonly with oral
TCA use can be avoided.

Opioids

The use of systemic opioids long has been a cornerstone of the treatment
of pain in those who have a terminal illness. Recently, the use of strong opioids in the treatment of pain not associated with malignancy has become
more mainstream but still is tinged with anxieties related to the systemic
effects of opioids, including tolerance and abuse.

It is becoming evident that opioid receptors are synthesized in dorsal root
ganglia and are transported into peripheral terminals of primary afferent
neurons [65,66]; μ- and δ-opioid receptors can be identified in fine cutaneous
nerves in opioid-naive animals [67]. These peripheral delta-opioid receptors
can be targeted experimentally with the δ-opioid receptor agonist loperamide, which does not cross the blood-brain barrier [68,69]. Many practitioners are familiar with the use of this drug in the treatment of diarrhea.
Further evidence of a peripheral opioid receptor presence is gained by the
fact that when a ligature is placed around the rat sciatic nerve, β-endorphin
binding sites accumulate proximally and distally to the ligature site [70].
When inflammation is induced, the number of β-endorphin binding sites
on both sides of the ligature increase massively [70].

A variety of reports suggests that topically applied morphine can reduce
pain from ulcers [71] and arthritic joints [72]. When used as an oral rinse, morphine can reduce mucositis-related pain in patients undergoing chemotherapy
for head and neck carcinomas [73,74], whereas intravesical treatment with
morphine can reduce painful bladder spasms [75,76]. Despite these suggestions, two systematic reviews failed to find any definitive proof of a pain-
relieving effect when morphine was used by peripheral application [77,78].

Therefore, although it is appealing to believe that those opioid receptors known to be present in the periphery could be targeted by local application of an opioid, in clinical practice, sound evidence for this effect is lacking.

á-Adrenoreceptor antagonists

Clonidine, an $á_2$-adrenoreceptor agonist, usually is administered by the oral route, although it can by given parenterally or by epidural injection. It also can be obtained in cream and patch formulations. It is likely that pain relief apparent after topical administration is the result of local and systemic actions. It is reported that clonidine patches reduce the hyperalgesia associated with sympathetically maintained pain but not in those who have sympathetically independent pain [79]. Clonidine cream also may have some pain-relieving effect in orofacial neuralgia-like pain [80]. The effect of clonidine in sympathetically maintained pain may be related to its effect of reducing presynaptic norepinephrine release from sympathetic nerves. When clonidine is injected into a knee joint after arthroscopy, pain relief may be observed [81,82]; when injected along with bupivicaine [83,84] and morphine [85], the analgesic effect of these drugs is enhanced.

Cannabinoids

Potential exists for the use of topically applied cannabinoids (CBs), because there are peripheral CB_1 and CB_2 receptors. When the animal formalin model [86], carrageenan hyperalgesia model [87], and nerve injury model [88] are examined, peripheral application of agents active on CB_1 receptors produces antinociception. This effect may be obtained because of the effects of these agents on the sensory nerve terminal to inhibit release of calcitonin gene-related peptide [87] or by inhibiting effects of nerve growth factor [89]. CB_2 receptor mechanisms may play a prominent role in inflammatory pain [89]. The clinical relevance of these findings is yet to be established firmly.

Glutamate receptors antagonists

Glutamate receptors are expressed on peripheral nerve terminals and these may contribute to peripheral nociceptive signaling. Ionotropic and metabotropic glutamate receptors are present on membranes of unmyelinated peripheral axons and axon terminals in the skin [90,91], and peripheral inflammation increases the proportions of unmyelinated and myelinated nerves expressing ionotropic glutamate receptors [92]. Local injections of NMDA and non-NMDA glutamate receptor agonists to the rat hind paw [93,94] or knee joint [95] enhance pain behaviors generating hyperalgesia and allodynia. Injections of metabotropic glutamate receptor agonists produce similar actions [90,96]. Local application of glutamate receptor antagonists inhibits pain behavior after formalin application [95].

In humans, ketamine, a noncompetitive NMDA receptor antagonist, enhances the local anesthetic and analgesic effects of bupivicaine in acute postoperative pain by a peripheral mechanism [97]. One study suggests that when a thermal injury was inflicted in volunteers, subcutaneous injection of ketamine produced long-lasting reduction in hyperalgesia [98], whereas a different study fails to confirm this result [99]. Not only may any analgesic effect produced by peripheral ketamine application be the result of its glutamate receptor activity but also ketamine may block voltage-sensitive calcium channels, alter cholinergic and monoaminergic actions, and interfere with opioid receptors [99–101].

Isolated case reports propose that topical ketamine can reduce sympathetically maintained pain [102] and pain of malignant origin [103,104], again suggesting that peripheral glutamate receptor antagonists may have an analgesic effect when applied topically.

Use of topical analgesics in elderly patients

Some perceive the use of the topical route of administration of a drug as a simplistic treatment. More certainty is present when a measured quantity of drug is given orally or when titrated intravenously. In the past, topical administration was believed somewhat "unscientific" and not worthy of medical attention or use. One thinks of the long-term availability of the topical NSAIDs and the reluctance of physicians to accept even that topical application of such drugs produced anything more than a placebo response. The weight of evidence confirming their pain-relieving effect from topical administration is substantial. Perhaps cynicism was promoted by a lack of understanding of the presence, or importance, of peripheral targets for topically applied analgesic agents. In addition, uncertainties about transdermal penetration of drugs made some of these therapeutic targets seem inaccessible, except when medication was administered systemically. Again, now it is known that many drugs are transferred efficiently across skin, and advances in technology have seen the production of "carriers" that enhance transdermal penetration.

In all patients, pharmacokinetic and pharmacodynamic factors control drug uptake and action. They also influence the risk for adverse effect heavily when drugs are administered. In a general sense, pharmacokinetic and pharmacodynamic changes in elderly patients increase the risk for such adverse effects. The likelihood of elderly patients taking other drugs with which a systemically administered analgesic could interact also is greater than in younger subjects. Therefore, if a localized pain can be targeted efficiently by use of a topical agent, where the risk for systemic uptake of that drug is low, then this seems to offer a significant advantage to any patient, in particular elderly patients whose ability to handle a systemic drug safely may be reduced.

It is suggested, therefore, that for example, the use of a topical nitrate rather than an oral NSAID over an arthritic joint or the use of a topical TCA or local anesthetic patch instead of an oral tricyclic or antiepileptic drug where patients have a localized neuropathic pain is a wise initial step in any elderly patient. Unfortunately, few of the topical analgesics discussed have an indication for the analgesic use outlined. Given the uncertainty of any company acquiring patent protection that would allow development of several of the topical options discussed previously, it is likely that their use will be occasional and not considered mainstream.

Taken as a whole, the topical agents discussed previously fall into several distinct groups. First are those for which there is substantial evidence of efficacy and that are available with a specific indication as topical analgesics—NSAIDs, local anesthetics, and capsaicin fall into this group. Second are those for which a body of clinical and preclinical evidence suggests that a topical analgesic effect is likely but for which no specific topical analgesic indication is in place. This include topical TCAs and nitrates. The last group comprises those agents in which the presence of peripheral receptors on which the drugs may work if applied topically are demonstrable and in which the evidence of a clinical effect is anecdotal at best. This last group includes opioids, CBs, á-adrenoreceptor antagonists, and the glutamate receptor antagonists.

Summary

Pain processing and transmission are achieved by a complex interaction of pathways and processes that stretch from the periphery to the central nervous system and back again. Those parts of this process that have peripheral representation may be amenable to therapeutic intervention by systemic administration of a drug to achieve a peripheral effect or by local application of a drug. This latter mode of therapy includes local topical administration of drug to the skin overlying the painful area. Among the advantages, particularly in elderly patients, are high level of patient acceptance, ease of administration, avoidance of systemic side effects of the drugs used, and reduced likelihood of drug-drug interactions.

Those drugs that have a known topical analgesic effect include those with a specific topical analgesic indication along with others in which, to date, no such indication exists but that may offer the chance of successful pain therapy at a reduced risk when compared with more conventional oral therapy.

References

[1] Mason L, Moore RA, Edwards JE, et al. Topical NSAIDs for acute pain: a meta-analysis. BMC Fam Pract 2004;5:10.
[2] Mazieres B. Topical ketoprofen patch. Drugs R D 2005;6:337–44.

[3] Ganerm-Quintanar A, Silva-Alvarez M, Alvarez-Roman R, et al. Design and evaluation of a self-adhesive naproxen-loaded film prepared from a nanoparticles dispersion. J Nanosci Nanotechnol 2006;6:3235–41.

[4] Alessandri F, Lijoi D, Mistrangelo E, et al. Topical diclofenac patch for postoperative would pain in laparoscopic gynecologic surgery: a randomized study. J Minim Invasive Gynecol 2006;13:195–200.

[5] Shaikh IM, Jadhav KR, Gide PS, et al. Topical delivery of aceclofenac from lecithin organogels: preformulation study. Curr Drug Deliv 2006;3:417–27.

[6] Heyneman CA, Lawless-Liday C, Wall GC. Oral versus topical NSAIDs in rheumatic diseases. A comparison. Drugs 2000;60:555–74.

[7] Vaile JI, Davis P. Topical NSAIDs for musculoskeletal conditions. A review of the literature. Drugs 1998;56:783–99.

[8] Galer BS. Topical medications. In: Loeser JD, editor. Bonica's management of pain. Philadelphia: Lippincott-Williams & Wilkins; 2001. p. 1736–41.

[9] Attal N, Brasseur L, Chauvin M. Effects of single and repeated applications of a eutectic mixture of local anesthetics (EMLA®) cream on spontaneous and evoked pain in post-herpetic neuralgia. Pain 1999;81:203–9.

[10] Litman SJ, Vitkun SA, Poppers PJ. Use of EMLA® cream in the treatment of post-herpetic neuralgia. J Clin Anesth 1996;8:54–7.

[11] Lycka BA, Watson CP, Nevin K, et al. EMLA® cream for the treatment of pain caused by post-herpetic neuralgia: a double-blind, placebo-controlled study. Proceedings of the Annual Meeting of the American Pain Society. Glenview (IL): American Pain Society; 1996. p. A111 [abstract].

[12] Rowbotham MC, Davis PS, Verkempinck C, et al. Lidocaine patch: double-blind controlled study of a new treatment method for post-herpetic neuralgia. Pain 1996;65: 39–44.

[13] Galer BS, Rowbotham MC, Perander J, et al. Topical lidocaine patch relieves post-herpetic neuralgia more effectively than vehicle patch: results of an enriched enrolment study. Pain 1999;80:533–8.

[14] Herrmann DN, Barbano RL, Hart-Gouleau S, et al. An open-label study of the lidocaine patch 5% in painful idiopathic sensory polyneuropathy. Pain Med 2005;6:379–84.

[15] Gammaitoni AR, Galer BS, Onawola R, et al. Lidocaine patch 5% and its positive impact on pain qualities in osteoarthritis: results of a pilot 2-week, open-label study using the Neuropathic Pain Scale. Curr Med Res Opin 2004;20(Suppl 2):S13–9.

[16] Fitzgerald M. Capsaicin and sensory neurones. Pain 1983;15:109–30.

[17] Rains C, Bryson HM. Topical capsaicin. A review of its pharmacological properties and therapeutic potential in postherpetic neuralgia, diabetic neuropathy and osteoarthritis. Drugs Aging 1995;7:317–28.

[18] Nolano M, Simone DA, Wendleschafer-Crabb G, et al. Topical capsaicin in humans: parallel loss of epidermal nerve fibers and pain sensation. Pain 1999;81:135–41.

[19] Tandan R, Lewis GA, Krusinski PB, et al. Topical capsaicin in painful diabetic neuropathy. Diabetes Care 1992;15:8–13.

[20] Capsaicin Study Group. Effect of treatment with capsaicin on daily activities of patients with painful diabetic neuropathy. Diabetes Care 1992;15:159–65.

[21] Chad DA, Aronin N, Lundstorm R, et al. Does capsaicin relieve pain of diabetic neuropathy? Pain 1990;42:387–8.

[22] Berstein JE, Korman NJ, Bickers DR, et al. Topical capsaicin treatment of chronic postherpetic neuralgia. J Am Acad Dermatol 1989;21:265–70.

[23] Watson CP, Tyler KL, Bickers DR, et al. A randomized vehicle controlled trial of topical capsaicin in the treatment of postherpetic neuralgia. Clin Ther 1993;15:510–26.

[24] Watson CP, Evans R, Watt VR. Post herpetic neuralgia and topical capsaicin. Pain 1988; 33:333–40.

[25] Low PA, Opfer-Gehrking TL, Dyck PJ, et al. Double blind, placebo controlled study of the application of capsaicin cream in chronic distal painful polyneuropathy. Pain 1995;45: 163–8.

[26] Morgenlander JC, Hurwitz BJ, Massey EW. Capsaicin for the treatment of pain in Guillain-Barré syndrome. Ann Neurol 1990;28:199.

[27] Epstein JB, Marcoe JH. Topical application of capsaicin for treatment of oral neuropathic pain and trigeminal neuralgia. Oral Surg Oral Med Oral Pathol 1994;77:135–40.

[28] Altman RD, Aven A, Holmberg CE, et al. Capsaicin cream 0.025% as monotherapy for osteoarthritis: a double blind study. Clinical Therapeutics 1994;23S:25–33.

[29] Deal CL. The use of topical capsaicin in managing arthritis pain: a clinician's perspective. Seminars in Arthritis and Rheumatism 1994;23S:48–52.

[30] Deal CL, Schnitzer TJ, Lipstein E, et al. Treatment of arthritis with topical capsaicin: a double blind trial. Clin Ther 1991;13:383–95.

[31] McCarthy GM, McCarty DJ. Effect of topical capsaicin in the therapy of painful osteoarthritis of the hands. J Rheumatol 1992;19:604–7.

[32] McCleane GJ. The analgesic efficacy of topical capsaicin is enhanced by glyceryl trinitrate in painful osteoarthritis: a randomised, double-blind, placebo-controlled study. Eur J Pain 2000;4:355–60.

[33] Schnitzer T, Morton C, Coker S. Topical capsaicin therapy for osteoarthritis: achieving a maintenance regimen. Seminars in Arthritis and Rheumatism 1994;23S:34–40.

[34] Mathias BJ, Dillingham TR, Zeigler DN, et al. Topical capsaicin for chronic neck pain. Am J Phys Med Rehabil 1995;74:39–44.

[35] Poyhia R, Vainio A. Topically administered ketamine reduces capsaicin-evoked mechanical hyperalgesia. Clin J Pain 2006;22:32–6.

[36] Yosipovitch G, Mailback HI, Rowbotham MC. Effect of EMLA pre-treatment on capsaicin-induced burning and hyperalgesia. Acta Derm Venereol 1999;79:118–21.

[37] Walker RA, McCleane GJ. The addition of glyceryl trinitrate to capsaicin cream reduces the thermal allodynia associated with the use of capsaicin alone in humans. Neurosci Lett 2002;323:78–80.

[38] McCleane GJ, McLaughlin M. The addition of GTN to capsaicin cream reduces the discomfort associated with application of capsaicin alone. Pain 1998;78:149–51.

[39] Feelisch M, Noack EA. Correlation between nitric oxide formation during degradation of organic nitrates and activation of guanylate cyclase. Eur J Pharmacol 1987;139: 19–30.

[40] Knowles RG, Palacios M, Palmer RM, et al. Formation of nitric oxide from L-arginine in the central nervous system: a transduction mechanism for stimulation of soluble guanylate cyclase. Proc Natl Acad Sci U S A 1989;86:159–62.

[41] Duarte ID, Lorenzetti BB, Ferreira SH. Acetylcholine induces peripheral analgesia by the release of nitric oxide. In: Moncada S, Higgs A, editors. Nitric oxide from L-arginine. A bio-regulatory system. Amsterdam: Elsevier; 1990. p. 165–70.

[42] Soares S, Leite R, Patsuo M, et al. Activation of ATP sensitive K channels: mechanisms of peripheral antinociceptive action of the nitric oxide donor, sodium nitroprusside. Eur J Pharmacol 2000;14:67–71.

[43] Paoloni JA, Appleyard RC, Nelson J, et al. Topical glyceryl trinitrate application in the treatment of chronic supraspinatus tendinopathy: a randomized, double-blinded, placebo-controlled clinical trial. Am J Sports Med 2005;33:806–13.

[44] Berrazueta JR, Losada A, Poveda J, et al. Successful treatment of shoulder pain syndrome due to supraspinatus tendonitis with transdermal nitroglycerin. A double blind study. Pain 1996;66:63–7.

[45] McCleane GJ. The addition of piroxicam to topically applied glyceryl trinitrate enhances the analgesic effect in musculoskeletal pain: a randomised, double-blind, placebo-controlled study. The Pain Clinic 2000;12:113–6.

[46] Berrazueta JR, Poveda JJ, Ochotoco JA, et al. The anti-inflammatory and analgesic action of transdermal glyceryl trinitrate in the treatment of infusion related thrombophlebitis. Postgrad Med J 1993;69:37–40.

[47] Berrazueta JR, Fleitas M, Salas E, et al. Local transdermal glyceryl trinitrate has an anti-inflammatory action on thrombophlebitis induced by sclerosis of leg varicose veins. Angiology 1994;45:347–51.

[48] Walsh KE, Berman JR, Berman LA, et al. Safety and efficacy of topical nitroglycerin for treatment of vulvar pain in women with vulvodynia: a pilot study. J Gend Specif Med 2002;5:21–7.

[49] Sawynok J. Adenosine receptor activation and nociception. Eur J Pharmacol 1998;317: 1–11.

[50] Esser MJ, Sawynok MJ. Caffeine blockade of the thermal antihyperalgesic effect of acute amitriptyline in a rat model of neuropathic pain. Eur J Pharmacol 2000;399:131–9.

[51] Sudoh Y, Cahoon EE, Garner P, et al. Tricyclic antidepressants as long acting local anesthetics. Pain 2003;103:49–55.

[52] Harder A, Gerner P, Kao G, et al. Cutaneous analgesia after transdermal application of amitriptyline versus lidocaine in rats. Anesth Analg 2003;96:1707–10.

[53] Esser MJ, Sawynok J. Acute amitriptyline in a rat model of neuropathic pain: differential symptom and route effects. Pain 1999;80:643–53.

[54] Esser MJ, Chase T, Allen GV, et al. Chronic administration of amitriptyline and caffeine in a rat model of neuropathic pain: multiple interactions. Eur J Pharmacol 2001;430:211–8.

[55] Sawynok J, Esser MJ, Reid AR. Peripheral antinociceptive actions of desipramine and fluoxetine in an inflammatory and neuropathic pain test in the rat. Pain 1999;82:149–58.

[56] Sawynok J, Reid AR, Esser MJ. Peripheral antinociceptive action of amitriptyline in the rat formalin test: involvement of adenosine. Pain 1999;80:45–55.

[57] Sawynok J, Reid A. Peripheral interactions between dextromethorphan, ketamine and amitriptyline on formalin-evoked behaviours and paw edema in rats. Pain 2003;102:179–86.

[58] Heughan CE, Allen GV, Chase TD, et al. Peripheral amitriptyline suppresses formalin-induced Fos expression in the rat spinal cord. Anesth Analg 2002;94:427–31.

[59] Su X, Gebhart GF. Effects of tricyclic antidepressants on mechanosensitive pelvic nerve afferent fibers innervating the rat colon. Pain 1998;76:105–14.

[60] Oatway M, Reid A, Sawynok J. Peripheral antihyperalgesic and analgesic actions of ketamine and amitriptyline in a model of mild thermal injury in the rat. Anesth Analg 2003;97:168–73.

[61] McCleane GJ. Topical doxepin hydrochloride reduces neuropathic pain: a randomized, double-blind, placebo controlled study. The Pain Clinic 1999;12:47–50.

[62] McCleane GJ. Topical administration of doxepin hydrochloride, capsaicin and a combination of both produces analgesia in chronic human neuropathic pain: a randomised, double-blind, placebo-controlled study. Br J Clin Pharmacol 2000;49:574–9.

[63] McCleane GJ. Topical application of doxepin hydrochloride can reduce the symptoms of complex regional pain syndrome: a case report. Injury 2002;33:88–9.

[64] Epstein JB, Truelove EL, Oien H, et al. Oral topical doxepin rinse: analgesic effect in patients with oral mucosal pain due to cancer or cancer therapy. Oral Oncol 2001;37:632–7.

[65] Zhou L, Zang Q, Stein C, et al. Contribution of opioid receptors on primary afferent versus sympathetic neurons to peripheral opioid analgesia. J Pharmacol Exp Ther 1998;286:1000–6.

[66] Stein C, Schafer M, Hassan AH. Peripheral opioid receptors. Ann Med 1995;27:219–21.

[67] Coggeshall RE, Zhou S, Carlton SM. Opioid receptors on peripheral sensory axons. Brain Res 1997;764:126–32.

[68] Shinoda K, Hruby VJ, Porreca F. Antihyperalgesic effects of loperamide in a model of rat neuropathic pain are mediated by peripheral delta-opioid receptors. Neurosci Lett 2007; 411:143–6.

[69] Shannon HE, Lutz EA. Comparison of the peripheral and central effects of the opioid agonists loperamide and morphine in the formalin test in rats. Neuropharmacology 2002;42:253–61.

[70] Hassan AH, Ableitner A, Stein C, et al. Inflammation of the rat paw enhances axonal transport of opioid receptors in the sciatic nerve and increases their density in the inflamed tissue. Neuroscience 1993;55:185–95.

[71] Zeppetella G, Paul J, Ribeiro MD. Analgesic efficacy of morphine applied topically to painful ulcers. J Pain Symptom Manage 2005;30:304–5.

[72] Wilken M, Ineck JR, Rule AM. Chronic arthritis pain management with topical morphine: case series. J Pain Palliat Care Pharmacother 2005;19:39–44.

[73] Cerchietti LC, Navigante AH, Bonomi MR, et al. Effect of topical morphine for mucositis-associated pain following concomitant chemoradiotherapy for head and neck carcinoma. Cancer 2002;95:2230–6.

[74] Cerchietti LC, Navigante AH, Körte MW, et al. Potential utility of the peripheral analgesic properties of morphine in stomatitis-related pain: a pilot study. Pain 2003;105:265–73.

[75] Duckett JW, Cangiano T, Cubina M, et al. Intravesical morphine analgesia after bladder surgery. J Urol 1997;157:1407–9.

[76] McCoubrie R, Jeffrey D. Intravesical diamorphine for bladder spasm. J Pain Symptom Manage 2003;25:1–2.

[77] Picard PR, Tramer MR, McQuay HJ, et al. Analgesic efficacy of peripheral opioids (all accept intra-articular): a quantitative systematic review of randomised controlled trials. Pain 1997;72:309–18.

[78] Gupta A, Bodin L, Holmstrom B, et al. A systematic review of the peripheral analgesic effects of intraarticular morphine. Anesth Analg 2001;93:761–70.

[79] Davis CL, Treede RD, Raja SN, et al. Topical application of clonidine relieves hyperalgesia in patients with sympathetically maintained pain. Pain 1991;47:309–17.

[80] Epstein JB, Grushka M, Le N. Topical clonidine for orofacial pain: a pilot study. J Orofac Pain 1997;11:346–52.

[81] Gentili M, Houssel P, Osman H, et al. Intra-articular morphine and clonidine produce comparable analgesia but the combination is not more effective. Br J Anaesth 1997;79:660–1.

[82] Gentili M, Juhel A, Bonnet F. Peripheral analgesic effect of intra-articular clonidine. Pain 1996;64:593–6.

[83] Reuben SS, Connelly NR. Postoperative analgesia for outpatient arthroscopic knee surgery with intra-articular clonidine. Anesth Analg 1999;88:729–33.

[84] Joshi M, Reuben SS, Kilaru PR, et al. Postoperative analgesia for outpatient arthroscopic knee surgery with intra-articular clonidine and/or morphine. Anesth Analg 2000;90:1102–6.

[85] Buerkle H, Huge V, Wolfgart M, et al. Intra-articular clonidine analgesia after knee arthroscopy. Eur J Anaesthesiol 2000;17:295–9.

[86] Calignano A, La Ranna G, Guiffrida A, et al. Control of pain initiation by endogenous cannabinoids. Nature 1998;394:277–81.

[87] Richardson JD, Kilo S, Hargreaves KM. Cannabinoids reduce hyperalgesia and inflammation via interaction with peripheral CB1 receptors. Pain 1998;75:111–9.

[88] Fox A, Kesingland A, Gentry C, et al. The role of central and peripheral cannabinoid1 receptors in the antihyperalgesic activity of cannabinoids in a model of neuropathic pain. Pain 2001;92:91–100.

[89] Rice AS, Farquhar-Smith WP, Nagy I. Endocannabinoids and pain: spinal and peripheral analgesia in inflammation and neuropathy. Prostaglandins Leukot Essent Fatty Acids 2002;66:243–56.

[90] Zhou S, Komak S, Du J, et al. Metabotropic glutamate 1α receptors on peripheral primary afferent fibres: their role in nociception. Brain Res 2001;913:18–26.

[91] Carlton SM, Hargett GL, Coggeshall RE. Localization and activation of glutamate receptors in unmyelinated axons of rat glabrous skin. Neurosci Lett 1995;197:25–8.

[92] Carlton SM, Coggeshall RE. Inflammation-induced changes in peripheral glutamate receptor populations. Brain Res 1999;820:63–70.

[93] Zhou S, Bonasera L, Carlton SM. Peripheral administration of NMDA, AMPA or KA results in pain behaviour in rats. Neuroreport 1996;7:895–900.

[94] Jackson DL, Graff CB, Richardson JD. Glutamate participates in the peripheral modulation of thermal hyperalgesia in rats. Eur J Pharmacol 1995;284:321–5.

[95] Lawland MB, Willis WD, Westlund KN. Excitatory amino acid receptor involvement in peripheral nociceptive transmission in rats. Eur J Pharmacol 1997;324:169–77.

[96] Walker K, Reeve A, Bowes M, et al. mGlu5 receptors and nociceptive function II. mGlu5 receptors functionally expressed on peripheral sensory neurones mediate inflammatory hyperalgesia. Neuropharmacology 2001;40:10–9.

[97] Tverskoy M, Oren M, Vaskovich M, et al. Ketamine enhances local anesthetic and analgesic effect of bupivicaine by a peripheral mechanism: a study in postoperative patients. Neurosci Lett 1996;215:5–8.

[98] Warncke T, Jórum E, Stubhaug A. Local treatment with the N-methyl-D-aspartate receptor antagonist ketamine inhibits development of secondary hyperalgesia in man by a peripheral action. Neurosci Lett 1997;227:1–4.

[99] Pedersen JL, Galle TS, Kehlet H. Peripheral analgesic effects of ketamine in acute inflammatory pain. Anesthesiology 1998;89:58–66.

[100] Hirota K, Lambert DG. Ketamine: its mechanism(s) of action and unusual clinical uses. Br J Anaesth 1996;77:441–4.

[101] Meller ST. Ketamine: relief from chronic pain through actions at the NMDA receptor? Pain 1996;68:435–6.

[102] Sawynok J, Reid MR. Modulation of formalin-induced behaviours and edema by local and systemic administration of dextromethorphan, memantine and ketamine. Eur J Pharmacol 2002;450:115–21.

[103] Crowley KL, Flores JA, Hughes CN, et al. Clinical application of ketamine ointment in the treatment of sympathetically maintained pain. International Journal Pharmaceutical Compounding 1998;2:122–7.

[104] Wood RM. Ketamine for pain in hospice patients. International Journal Pharmaceutical Compounding 2000;4:253–4.

ELSEVIER
SAUNDERS

CLINICS IN
GERIATRIC
MEDICINE

Clin Geriatr Med 24 (2008) 313–334

Role of Rehabilitation Medicine in the Management of Pain in Older Adults

Hyon Schneider, MD[a], Adrian Cristian, MD[b,c],*

[a]Department of Rehabilitation Medicine, The Mount Sinai Medical Center,
1425 Madison Avenue, Box 1240, New York, NY 10029-6574, USA
[b]Department of Rehabilitation Medicine, James J. Peters Veterans Affairs Medical Center,
Room 3d-16 526/117, 130 West Kingsbridge Road, Bronx, NY 10468, USA
[c]Department of Rehabilitation Medicine, Mount Sinai School of Medicine,
New York, NY, USA

According to the 2000 US Census, there are 35 million Americans over the age 65 [1]. With increasing life expectancy, the projected number of older persons will reach one in five Americans by the year 2030, a nearly fourfold increase from 100 years earlier. Along with increasing longevity, maintaining quality of life by preserving health, comfort, and physical function is a priority in the growing geriatric population. Quality of life may be affected significantly by pain and its impact on physical function and disabilities.

Pain management may play an important role in contributing to optimal quality of life in the elderly population. Pain lowers overall quality of life in part by decreasing function and by amplifying the psychological stress of aging. Pain can result in an older person being confined to their home and effectively isolate patients physically, socially, and emotionally. Pain must be treated early and effectively to preserve function and quality of life. A comprehensive, multidisciplinary approach to pain management, with preservation and restoration of function in older adults, is the cornerstone of an effective pain management program.

Although new onset or progression of diseases is common in older adults, pain is not a normal part of the aging process. The belief that pain is a normal part of the aging process is shared by many older adults and their significant others and can lead to under-reporting of pain, resulting in potential delays in treatment.

* Corresponding author. Department of Rehabilitation Medicine, James J Peters Veterans Affairs Medical Center, Room 3d-16 526/117, 130 West Kingsbridge Road, Bronx, NY 10468.
E-mail address: adrian.cristian@va.gov (A. Cristian).

Prevalence of pain in older adults

The prevalence of pain in the elderly averages roughly 50% in a community setting to almost 80% in institutional settings. The prevalence of pain in community-dwelling residents has been reported to be between 32.5% and 71.5%, with the most common locations being limb joints and back [2,3]. This is comparable to the prevalence rates of pain reported by residents of long-term care facilities, which has been reported to be between 45% and 80% [4–6].

Etiology of pain

The two leading causes of pain in the geriatric population are cancer and arthritis. Cancer is the most common cause of pain, with 30% to 40% prevalence in patients undergoing treatment and 70% to 90% prevalence in patients who have advanced disease [7].

Arthritis is the second most common cause of pain and a leading cause of disabilities in the United States. Approximately 60% of the United States population is affected by arthritis [8]. If this arthritis prevalence rate remains stable, the number of affected persons over the age of 65 will nearly double by 2030 [9,10]. Among those who had arthritis, 10% to 30% reported significant pain leading to disability [11]. The US Centers for Disease Control and Prevention (CDC) estimates that 12 million Americans will have functional limitations secondary to osteoarthritis (OA) by the year 2020 and are estimating close to $65 billion disability costs annually [11].

Other common causes of pain included acute inflammation, postherpetic neuralgia, low back pain secondary to degenerative changes in facet joints and discs, spinal stenosis, fibromyalgia, poststroke pain, and diabetic peripheral neuropathy.

Pain classifications

Pain can be classified by duration (chronic versus acute) or by its pathophysiology, as seen in Box 1.

Types of pain

There are two main types of pain: nociceptive and neuropathic. The following sections briefly describe both types of pain.

Nociceptive pain

Nociceptive pain can be acute or chronic. It typically is well localized, described as aching, squeezing, stabbing, or throbbing, and tends to respond well to opioids and anti-inflammatories. Examples of nociceptive pain

---

Box 1. Examples of acute and chronic pain

Acute pain
Acute inflammation
Infections
Skin ulcerations

Chronic pain
Osteoarthritis
Facet arthropathy
Spinal stenosis
Fibromyalgia
Poststroke pain
Diabetic neuropathy

---

include sprains, fractures, burns, bruises, inflammation from an infection or arthritis, bowel obstructions, and myofascial pain.

The nociceptive pain pathway has four processes: transduction, transmission, modulation, and perception.

Transduction

Tissue injury and accompanying inflammation/noxious stimuli depolarize peripheral nociceptors, which are lightly myelinated or nonmyelinated ends of primary afferent nociceptive sensory neurons.

Transmission

Nociceptors carry signals (by means of A-delta and C-fibers) to the dorsal horn of the spinal cord, where signals are relayed and cross over to contralateral ascending fibers. These fibers carry signals to the thalamus and the cortex, including the postcentral gyrus in the brain.

Modulation

Other surrounding nociceptors may be activated and/or sensitized by the release of substance P, serotonin, histamine, acetylcholine, prostaglandins, and bradykinin. Prostaglandins produced at the site of injury may act to further enhance the nociceptive response to inflammation by lowering the threshold to noxious stimulation. Chronic inflammation with nociceptive stimulation may be the source of persistent pain. Analgesia is mediated in part by the binding of endogenous opioids to mu, delta, and kappa receptors.

Perception

Pain is perceived only when the impulses reach the brain. Therefore, the ultimate perception of pain depends on both activity in this afferent system and its modulation by neurotransmitters, such as endorphins, substance P, serotonin, and norepinephrine.

Neuropathic pain

Neuropathic pain often is localized poorly. It frequently is described as a continuous burning, electric shock-like, squeezing, lancinating pain with or without numbness and tingling. Neuropathic pain may be referred to other areas of the body. Some terms that commonly associated with neuropathic pain include:

Allodynia (pain with non-noxious stimuli, eg, light touch)
Hyperalgesia (extreme sensitivity to response to noxious stimuli)
Hyperpathia (a painful syndrome characterized by an abnormally painful sensation to a stimulus, especially with a repetitive stimulus and/or an increased threshold) [12]

Neuropathic pain is frequently chronic and tends to have a poorer response to opioid treatment than nociceptive pain. Neuropathic pain processes may not be fully reversible, but partial improvement is often possible with proper treatment such as antiseizure (antiepileptic) and antidepressant medications.

Some examples of neuropathic pain include: postherpetic neuralgia, complex regional pain syndrome (CRPS), phantom limb pain, spinal cord injury pain, poststroke central pain, brachial plexopathy, cervical radiculopathy, entrapment neuropathy (eg, carpal tunnel syndrome), and peripheral neuropathies (associated with diabetes, chronic alcohol use, toxins, chemotherapies, and vitamin deficiencies).

Neuropathic pain is the result of an injury or malfunction in the peripheral or central nervous system. Injury to the nerve can be caused by: trauma (laceration or traction), nerve infiltrated or compressed by tumors, nerve strangulated by scar or fibrous tissue, or nerve inflamed by infection or autoimmune disorders.

Abnormal nerve regeneration can result following the initial injury to the peripheral axons in the ensuing weeks to months. The damaged axon may grow multiple nerve sprouts, some of which may form neuromas. Unlike normal axons, these structures can generate spontaneous activity and are more sensitive to physical distention. This is associated clinically with a positive Tinel's sign (a sensation of tingling or pins and needles in the distribution of the nerve upon percussion over the nerve).

Abnormal connections also may develop between new nerve sprouts and demyelinated axons in the region of the nerve damage, permitting abnormal communication between somatic or sympathetic efferent nerves and nociceptors [13].

Physical medicine and rehabilitation approach to pain management

The goals of rehabilitation medicine in the pain management of the older adult are to reduce pain, maximize function, and decrease disability.

To accomplish these goals, a multidisciplinary team approach often is used. Depending on the setting, this team can consist of a physiatrist (physician specializing in physical medicine and rehabilitation), physical therapist, occupational therapist, pain psychologist, rehabilitation nurse, recreational therapist, nutritionist, and social worker. All clinicians performs their own evaluations and establishes goals specific to their discipline based on the need of the patient. Timelines are set in which these goals can be met, and progress toward these goals is monitored at regular intervals (usually monthly). Once goals are met, either new goals are set, or the patient is discharged from the program with a home program. Depending on the complexity of the pain and its impact on the older individual, the care can be rendered in an inpatient or outpatient setting with appropriate additional consultants (ie, psychiatrist, surgeon, geriatrician...) called in as necessary.

Roles of rehabilitation medicine clinicians in pain management of the older adult

Physiatrist

The physiatrist, is a physician trained in physical medicine and rehabilitation who often treats pain secondary to painful conditions of the nervous and musculoskeletal systems by using medications, injections, exercise therapy, and orthotics. He or she also is trained in electrodiagnostic medicine and can perform electrodiagnostic tests that can be used to diagnose painful conditions such as radiculopathies and entrapment neuropathies such as carpal tunnel syndrome.

The physiatrist also can coordinate the care rendered by the various clinicians involved in the care of the older adult with pain.

Physical therapist

The role of the physical therapist is in both the evaluation and treatment of a patient's pain condition. The evaluation typically focuses on impairments of the nervous and musculoskeletal systems such as loss of range of motion in joints and spine, muscle strength deficiencies, and functional deficits relating to balance and ambulation. The treatment often consists of a combination of judicious use of modalities (heat, cold, electrical stimulation) and progressive exercises to strengthen weakened muscles and improve balance [14].

Occupational therapist

The role of the occupational therapist (OT) in the care of the older adult who has pain focuses on two broad areas—impairments in the upper extremities and functional losses due to pain—that affect the older adult's everyday life. The OT performs an evaluation of the nervous and musculoskeletal system with a special emphasis on range of motion, muscle strength, and fine motor control in the upper extremities.

The treatment often consists of a combination of modalities (ie, heat packs, fluidotherapy, paraffin, ultrasound), exercises, and upper extremity orthotics. Because painful conditions also can affect the older adult's ability to perform activities of daily living, the OT can make recommendations on devices that can make it easier and safer to carry out such activities (eg, sock-aids, hand-held reachers, tub benches, grab bars, hand held showers...).

Psychologist

Pain psychology assessment and therapeutic interventions focus on cognitive and behavioral factors related to pain. Psychological intervention in pain management of the elderly population focuses on unlearning or preventing maladaptive responses and reactions to pain while fostering self-efficacy, wellness, perceived control, and improved coping skills. Psychologists can help patients with pain by teaching them various coping strategies [15–17]. Some patients even with the best efforts of experts may continue to experience pain, and psychologists are a great asset in helping patients adjust to persistent pain by self-efficacy, pain coping strategies, readiness to change, and acceptance [17]. As a member of the rehabilitation team, the psychologist also assists other team members when psychological issues complicate efforts to provide effective pain management therapy.

Nurse

The role of rehabilitation nurses in an outpatient setting is related largely to patient education, documentation compliance, and liaisons with physiatrists. Nursing staff play an essential role in educational aspects of treatment, including basic instruction on pain pathways, pharmacology, nutrition, and sleep hygiene. In inpatient settings, rehabilitation nurses also serve as patient advocates in ongoing communication with all team members [18].

Therapeutic recreation counselor

Therapeutic recreation specialists evaluate and plan leisure activities for the promotion of mental and physical health. They help patients establish and integrate the functional and cognitive behavioral pain management strategies learned from other disciplines of treatments into social and community situations. Techniques incorporated from other disciplines include biomechanical and postural correction, pacing, and relaxation strategies.

Social worker

Social workers can provide counseling to patients and families regarding emotional support, community resources, finances, lifestyle changes, and participation in treatment. In some outpatient settings, social workers lead support groups, while in inpatient settings, they actively assist in discharge planning.

Common rehabilitation interventions for the treatment of pain in older adults

Rehabilitation medicine has an integral role in the treatment of painful conditions that affect older adults such as OA (shoulders, hips, knees, spine), tendonitis, bursitis, and radiculopathy (cervical and lumbar).

There are five main treatments rendered by rehabilitation medicine professionals for the treatment of pain:

Medications (ie, nonsteroidal anti-inflammatory drugs [NSAIDs], anti-epileptics, opiates...)
Modalities (ie, heat, cold, electrical stimulation)
Exercises (ie, muscle strengthening, balance)
Injections (ie, peripheral joints, trigger point)
Orthotic prescriptions

Some of these interventions are described briefly in the following sections.

Modalities

Modalities can be effective in the reduction of acute and chronic pain. Acute musculoskeletal pain is associated with an increase in local blood flow, release of inflammatory agents, and edema. Physical modalities such as cryotherapy (eg, cold packs) can reduce local edema and blood flow and thereby reduce pain (Table 1). Chronic musculoskeletal pain caused by OA may respond to heat modalities by relaxing local muscles that surround painful joints (Table 2). Electrical stimulation may be associated with a release of endorphins (Table 3) that aid in pain reduction.

Modalities are most effective when used in combination with exercise, patient education, medications, and/or interventional procedures. Some modalities also may be prescribed for home use. Patients are educated on pain prevention, home exercises, and proper use of physical agents at home [19]. There are various different physical agents/techniques available in major therapeutic categories of heat therapy, cryotherapy, and electrotherapy, each with specific physiologic effects that are described in Box 2.

Selections in types and settings of modalities for the treatment of pain are based on diagnosis, etiology of pain, anatomic location/target tissue, and careful consideration of contraindications.

Massage

Massage therapy can be of benefit to older adults who have painful conditions of the musculoskeletal system. There are several different types of massage therapy including Swedish, shiatsu, and acupressure; however, the exact mechanism of action is not known fully. It may work by increasing

Table 1
Cryotherapy agents

Physical agents	Description	Indication	Contraindication
Ice massage:	Ice is stroked gently on painful area.	General use of cryotherapy:	General contraindications of cryotherapy:
Cryocompression unit:	Sleeves with circulating cold water with pneumatic compression (60 mm Hg) at 7.2°C applied to affected limb	Acute/chronic pain: Sprains Strains Tendonitis Tenosynovitis Bursitis Adhesive capsulitis Myofascial	Impaired sensation Application >30 min Ischemia Arterial insufficiency Raynaud's disease Cryoglobulinemia Cold intolerance
Vapocoolant spray:	Fluori-methane spray or ethyl chloride	Acute injury with inflammation and edema in first 24 to 48 hrs Osteoarthritis Minor burns Spasticity	Severe cardiac or respiratory disease Cognitive or communication deficits that preclude reporting of pain

Adapted from Perret DM, Rim J, Cristian A. A geriatrician's guide to the use of physical modalities in the treatment of pain and dysfunction. Clin Geriatr Med 2006;22:331–54; with permission.

local blood flow, local temperature, releasing of endorphins, and serving as a counterirritant to the skin or inducing a generalized sense of relaxation. Massage therapy is contraindicated over local cancers, skin infections, areas of local trauma, or in limbs with known deep vein thrombosis [20].

Therapeutic exercise

Therapeutic exercise plays an important role in pain prevention and alleviation by preserving or restoring proper function in the affected areas. This is accomplished through various exercises that maximize range of movement, improve flexibility, increase muscle strength in muscles that stabilize painful joints, build cardiovascular endurance, and correct maladaptive antalgic movement patterns. Daily exercise has been associated with 25% less self-reported musculoskeletal pain in active versus sedentary participants in a 14-year prospective, longitudinal study [21]. Inactivity also has been shown to be a predictor of future pain and injury [22]. A brief description of the different types of exercises commonly used follows.

Range of motion exercise

A full range of motion (ROM) across a joint is very important to its proper function. ROM exercises help patients to regain as much movement

Table 2
Heat modalities

Physical agents	Description	Indication	Contraindication
Heating pads	Electrical heating pads or circulating fluid or gel filled packs Peak temp: 52°C (125° F)	General use of heat Pain in: Neck, Low back	General heat contraindications: Acute trauma Impaired sensation
Hydrocollator	Canvas filled with silicon dioxide immersed in tanks at 74.5°C (166° F) Applied over a moist towel	Myofascial Neuromas Pain secondary to: Tendonitis	Impaired circulation Acute inflammation Bleeding disorders Edema
Paraffin baths	Paraffin wax and mineral oil heated mixture of 6:1 or 7:1 ratio at temperature 52.2 to 54.4°C (126 to 130° F) Typically applied to hand by: 1. Dipping hand: 7–12 dips; then wrap in plastic and towels or insulating mitt. 2. Immersion: several dips to form a thin glove layer then immersion for 30 min 3. Brushing: brush on several coats then cover with towel.	Tenosynovitis Bursitis Muscle spasms Chronic inflammation Strains Sprains Joint stiffness Contractures	Large scars Local malignancy Atrophic skin Cognitive or communication deficits that preclude reporting of pain Poor thermal regulation Metallic prosthetic implants
Fluidotherapy	Dry heat modality: forced hot air through a bed of finely divided solid particles Massage action of the turbulence of the air blown particles 46.1 to 48.9°C (115 to 120° F)		
Infrared lamps	Molecular vibration, maximum radiation when perpendicular to surface		
Ultrasound	Sound waves used to generate heat Deep heat modality: 4–5°C elevation in temperature at depths of 8 cm	Bursitis Tendonitis Musculoskeletal pain Degenerative arthritis Joint contractures Hip contractures Adhesive capsulitis Subacute trauma Morton's neuroma	General heat contraindications In addition, avoid using ultrasound over: Brain Cervical ganglia Spine Laminectomy sites Near eyes Arthroplasties Reproductive organs Gravid uterus Menstruating uterus Near pacemaker Near tumors Skeletal immaturity
Phonophoresis	Use of ultrasound to facilitate transdermal Delivery of topical medication such as corticosteroids	Soft tissue inflammation	General heat contraindications

Adapted from Perret DM, Rim J, Cristian A. A geriatrician's guide to the use of physical modalities in the treatment of pain and dysfunction. Clin Geriatr Med 2006;22:331–54; with permission.

Table 3
Electrotherapy (electrical stimulation)

Physical agents	Description	Indication	Contraindication
TENS (transcutaneous electrical nerve stimulation)	Battery-operated device that delivers low-intensity electrical current through adhesive pads placed on the skin surface.	Pain management: Acute and chronic musculoskeletal pain Chronic neurogenic pain Peripheral nerve injury	Sensory impairment Circulatory impairment Arterial/venous thrombosis Thrombophlebitis Simulation over the
Iontophoresis	Use of electrical current to aid in delivery of medications to the target area driving across the skin	Peripheral neuropathy Phantom limb pain Post-traumatic pain Sympathetically mediated pain Postherpetic neuralgia Joint effusion Muscle disuse atrophy Circulatory disorders Venous insufficiency Neurovascular disorders Osteoarthritis Rheumatoid arthritis Dermal ulcers, wounds	carotid sinus Stimulation across the heart Near pacemaker Pregnancy Seizure disorder Fresh fracture Active hemorrhage Malignancy Atrophic skin Impaired cognition Known allergies to gel or pads

as possible in the affected joint. They usually are started before a muscle strengthening program.

There are three types of ROM exercises: passive, active, and active assisted. In passive ROM (PROM) exercises, the therapist moves the affected limb without any assistance from the patient. In active assisted ROM (AAROM) exercises, the patient provides some effort, and the treating therapist assists in the movement of the affected limb. In active ROM (AROM) exercises, the patient moves the affected body part on his/her own.

Strengthening exercises

Painful body parts such as the spine and extremities can be associated with limited use because of pain. This can lead to atrophy of the muscles that provide structural support to that body part. Strengthening the muscles around a joint helps to stabilize it, which in turn can reduce pain and prevent further injury. Muscle strength is affected by the type of muscle fibers contracting, the speed of contraction, the cross-sectional size of the muscle, the length–tension relationship, and the recruitment of motor units. The goal of a muscle strengthening program is to increase the maximal force that a muscle or muscle group can generate [23,24].

Muscle strengthening can be achieved in several ways: increasing the amount of weight lifted, increasing the speed of each contraction, or increasing the total number of contractions.

Box 2. Some physiologic effects of modalities

Physiologic effects of heat
Decrease pain
General relaxation
Increased acute inflammation
Increased edema–acute injury
Increase nerve conduction velocity
Increased blood flow and bleeding
Vasodilation of blood vessels
Increase tendon extensibility
Decrease joint stiffness
Increase in collagen elasticity and collagenase activity
Cutaneous counter-irritant effect
Release of endorphins

Physiologic effects of cold
Decrease pain
General relaxation
Decrease acute inflammation
Decrease nerve conduction velocity (motor and sensory)
Decrease muscle spindle activity (Ia and II)
Decrease muscle fatigue
Decrease muscle spasm and spasticity
Decrease metabolism
Decrease collagenase activity
Decrease elasticity
Increase viscosity
Increase joint stiffness

Physiologic effects of transcutaneous electrical nerve stimulation
Muscle group contraction
Slows muscle atrophy
Increases muscle strength
Increases circulation
Decreases muscle spasm
Increased release of endorphins
Promotes wound healing
Induces osteogenesis
Inhibits pain fibers: stimulates large myelinated type A nerve fibers (gate control theory)

Adapted from Perret DM, Rim J, Cristian A: A geriatrician's guide to the use of physical modalities in the treatment of pain and dysfunction. Clin Geriatr Med 2006;22:331–54.

Increased muscle strength within the initial 6 weeks of exercise results from the improved efficiency in motor unit recruitment process, a neuromuscular adaptation. Motor unit recruitment efficiency improves by recruiting larger motor units with higher frequencies of stimulation to generate force necessary to overcome the imposed resistance.

Following the initial neuromuscular adaptation, muscle hypertrophy takes place after 6 to 7 weeks of resistance training [25,26]. Muscle hypertrophy is the increased total muscle mass and cross-sectional area. A muscle's ability to produce force is directly proportional to its cross-sectional area. There are three different mechanisms that lead to muscle hypertrophy: increase in the number of myofibrils, muscle fiber hyperplasia, and new sarcomere formation.

Almost all muscle hypertrophy results from an increase in the number of myofibrils within a muscle fiber. New myofibrils are formed by splitting of the existing ones. In contrast, less than 5% of muscle hypertrophy is caused by the fiber hyperplasia (an increase in the number of muscle fibers) [25].

Another type of muscle hypertrophy can result from adding new sarcomeres at the muscle fibers ends, where they attach to the tendons. This occurs when muscle is stretched to greater than its normal length. Hence, ROM exercises contribute to muscle strengthening through the formation of new sarcomeres [26].

Muscle fibers characteristics

Muscle fibers are categorized based on speed of contraction—slow versus fast (Table 4). Muscle hypertrophy is more common in fast-twitch than slow-twitch muscles. Type 2A fibers exhibit the greatest growth, more so than type 2B and type 1 fibers.

Muscle contractions are categorized by: changes in length during contraction (concentric, eccentric) and the force applied to the muscle during the contraction (isometric, isotonic and isokinetic).

A concentric muscle contraction refers to a shortening of a muscle whereas an eccentric muscle contraction refers to a lengthening of a muscle.

Table 4
Types of muscle fibers

Slow-twitch Fibers	Fast-twitch Fibers	
Type 1	Type 2A	Type 2B
Slow oxidative, aerobic metabolism, high in oxidative enzymes and rich in capillary supply	Fatigue resistant, fast oxidative-glycolytic, higher level of oxidative enzymes and capillary supply (has some properties of type 1 fibers)	Fatigue easily glycolytic
Endurance activities	Strength and speed activities	Strength and speed activities

Both isotonic and isokinetic muscle contractions involve changes in muscle length (concentrically or eccentrically) and visible limb movement. In an isometric muscle contraction, the muscle length remains constant. An isotonic muscle contraction is performed at variable speed opposing a constant external resistance, whereas an isokinetic muscle contraction is performed at a constant velocity against a constant external angular velocity (variable external resistance).

Aerobic exercises

The purpose of an aerobic exercise program is to improve cardiovascular endurance. This is accomplished through exercises that involve large muscle groups in the upper and lower extremities by means of activities such as walking, running, swimming, and cycling.

Aerobic exercises are low-intensity, high-repetition, high-resistance, short-duration exercises at 60% to 80% of maximum exertion capacity. Physiologic effects of aerobic exercise include an increase in capillary density around the muscle fibers, increase in the number of mitochondria and their enzymatic activities, and increase in myoglobin content enhancing the energy supply to the muscles. Aerobic exercise also is associated with an increased level of endogenous endorphins [27] and enkephalins [28] that may contribute to the analgesic effect.

Balance exercise

Good balance depends on optimal muscle strength and proprioception in the trunk and lower extremities. Impaired proprioception has been associated with increased risk of joint damage and falls. Decreased joint proprioception is thought to influence the progressive joint deterioration associated with osteoarthritis and rheumatoid arthritis [29,30]. Several studies have shown that the risk of falling in the elderly population is correlated with postural sway, a variable that is determined in large part by proprioception [31–34]. Proprioception decreases with age, neuropathies, injuries, and underlying diseases such as diabetic neuropathy, osteoarthritis, rheumatoid arthritis, or trauma to knee and/or ankle ligaments.

Balance can be impaired in older adults who have coexisting disabilities such as stroke and painful hip osteoarthritis. Balance exercises are a combination of lower extremity strengthening exercises in key muscle groups (ie, illiopsoas, gluteus maximus, gluteus medius, quadriceps, gastrocnemius and anterior tibialis) along with proprioceptive exercises such as standing on one limb, standing on a tilt board, sideways/backward walking, and heel-to-toe walking that progressively challenge the patient's center of gravity in both static and dynamic positions. The purpose of proprioceptive exercises is to improve joint and limb position sense.

Exercise prescription

The exercise prescription typically is made up of the following components:

Precautions (ie, cardiac, pulmonary, falls, weight bearing status, infectious)
Type of exercise program (ie, range of motion, strengthening, cardiovascular)
Intensity of exercise (ie, number of repetitions, amount of weight to be lifted)
Duration of exercise (ie, cardiovascular—30 minutes per day, four to five times per week)
Rate of progression of exercise program (ie, increase weight by 10% every week)
Goals to be accomplished in a specific time frame

Injections

Injections are used commonly by physiatrists for managing painful conditions of the musculoskeletal system. Joints, periarticular structures, and muscles can be injected for therapeutic purposes. In addition to reducing pain, injections can facilitate participation in exercise programs that can help with regaining lost motion, improving strength of adjacent muscles, and improving function. A brief description of some commonly used injections follows.

Corticosteroid injections

Glucocorticosteroids often are mixed with a local anesthetic in injections for treating pain from inflammatory processes [35]. Selection of corticosteroids should be based on the size and tissue composition of the site of injection and the characteristics of the corticosteroid. It is important to know the differences among the different corticosteroids available and their contraindications. Available corticosteroids vary in strength and duration of action. For example, triamcinolone hexacetonide has the longest duration of suppression of inflammatory activity. Adverse effects such as infections, tissue atrophy, skin discoloration, elevated glucose levels, and elevated blood pressure should be explained to patients and discussed with their primary care physician. There is also an increased risk of pneumothorax with injection of soft tissues over the posterior thorax and an increased risk of local bleeding in patients on anticoagulation therapy.

Following the injection, the patient should be counseled on limiting activities involving the injected region, application of ice, and self-monitoring for signs of infection. The patient also should be told that there may be some local soreness of the injected region [36].

Local anesthetic injection

Local anesthetic injection in a perineural fashion may produce a transient block of ion flux through the axon's sodium channels, thereby halting conduction of impulses. Blocking the transmission from the peripheral nerves prevents input to the central nervous system. The degree of a nerve block depends on the properties of the anesthetic agent and the way in which it was administered [35].

Hyaluronate intra-articular injection

Sodium hyaluronate (ie, hyaluronan) has been shown to be a safe and effective treatment for the symptomatic relief of knee OA. HA may act as a shock absorber and lubricant to the joint. Intra-articularly injected HA is a viscoelastic supplement that is thought to essentially replace the diseased synovial fluid of the osteoarthritic joint [37]. Sodium hyaluronate is a natural substance derived from chicken comb and is similar to the synovial fluid of healthy young persons [38]. Studies demonstrate that this compound reduces joint pain for 1 week to 1 year in most patients [37,38]. The largest meta-analysis of 76 controlled clinical studies using intra-articular HAs was published recently and updated by the Cochrane Collaboration. This class of therapy was concluded to be effective and safe in patients who have knee osteoarthritis [39].

The exact mechanism of action for HA's role in pain relief remains unknown. Some explanations, however, include:

A role as a mechanical barrier to the activation of nociceptors
Inhibition of pain mediators such as prostaglandin e_2 and bradykinin
Anti-inflammatory effect by means of inhibition of cytokines
Increased endogenous production of hyaluronate by the joint
Restoration of physical characteristics of the synovial fluid [37]

There are five US Food and Drug Administration (FDA) approved intra-articular HAs for treating pain associated with knee OA. The medication is injected into the joint every week for either 3 weeks or 5 weeks. The most common adverse event of the HA intra-articular injection is injection site pain, which usually is remedied with a cold compress following the injection.

In general, this treatment should be reserved for those who have not responded to treatment with simple analgesics such as acetaminophen or to nonpharmacologic treatment (ie, physical therapy), and those who have radiographically demonstrable mild to moderate OA, and may have had a positive yet limited response to glucocorticoid injection. The drug is contraindicated in patients who have known hypersensitivity to it, and caution must be used in prescribing it for patients who have chicken allergies [37].

Myofascial trigger point injections

Myofascial pain originates in muscles and their fascial linings and often is associated with one or more trigger point(s). Trigger points are localized tender points in muscles with referred pain on palpation. They commonly are described as having a ropey, tense, and palpable band texture. Trigger points are found commonly in paraspinal muscles, but also can be present in the extremities and scalp.

When compared with equivalent palpation pressure applied in normal muscles, trigger points display focal hyperirritable palpable nodular areas located in a taut band of skeletal muscle with increased tenderness and a referred area of pain. Associated motor and/or autonomic dysfunction may be present [40].

The typically affected muscle is in a state of constant tension and is characterized by an inability to undergo full contraction and relaxation cycles. Sustained muscle contraction may lead to local vasoconstriction of myofascial tissue, which may result in a reduced oxygen tension, a build up of metabolic waste products, and the release of nociceptive chemicals in the muscle tissue.

Characteristic referral patterns include headaches, paresthesias, and various radiating symptoms. Characteristic referral patterns may be related to nociceptive sensory overload of the segmental dorsal root ganglion and dorsal horn of the spinal cord, resulting in overflow on a dermatomal, myotomal, radicular, or autonomic level [41].

Inadequate treatment of myofascial pain can result in an impaired posture, decreased range of motion, and decreased strength and decreased endurance.

Trigger point injections can be performed using various agents such as local anesthetics, steroids, saline, botulinum toxin, or dry needling of the affected points in muscles. Interestingly, in a recent review by Cumming and White, the therapeutic effect of trigger point injections did not depend on the agents injected. Local anesthetic, saline, or water were roughly equal in efficacy to dry needling techniques [42].

The injection is performed directly into the identified tender point. Following needle insertion, the needle is directed in a few directions, with small amounts of injected material delivered in each direction. Careful attention should be used when injecting in vascular areas, near nerves, or over the thorax. It is imperative that the clinician have experience and a very good working knowledge of the pertinent anatomy in the region being injected.

Trigger point injections are most useful when followed by passive stretch and in combination with therapy to promote maximum flexibility and strength.

Orthotics

An orthosis is defined as a device attached or applied to the external surface of the body to improve function, restrict, or enforce motion or support a body segment [43,44]. Orthotics play an important role in pain reduction and preservation of joints by providing proper joint mechanics and alignment. Orthotics stabilize joints and decrease joint motion and joint loading. They also provide support to the joint to allow maximal motion and function. Splints may be prefabricated or custom-molded.

Upper extremity orthotics for painful conditions in older adults

Orthotics for the wrist and hand are prescribed commonly for conditions such as carpal tunnel syndrome, rheumatoid arthritis, OA, and De Quervain's tenosynovitis. Their primary role is to protect and restrict painful movements of the wrist and fingers. Resting hand splints typically are worn during the daytime when the person is most active, but also can be worn during the night when nocturnal paresthesias may be present because of carpal tunnel syndrome.

Lower extremity orthotics for painful conditions in older adults

Lower limb orthotics are used to improve gait, reduce pain, decrease weight bearing, control movement, and minimize progression of a deformity. The most commonly prescribed orthotics for the lower extremities are for the knees, ankles, and feet. Ambulation aids (ie, walkers, canes, and crutches) can be used in combination with lower limb orthoses to help ensure safe mobility.

Foot orthoses

Excess pronation at the subtalar joint, loss of the medial arch, and subtalar movement are commonly seen foot deformities that also can cause pain and strain on the knee and hip. Control of pronation by bringing the calcaneus perpendicular to the floor often relieves pain. A hind foot orthotic has been shown to improve gait and reduce pain (Table 5) [41,45].

Lateral heel wedges are generally effective in alleviating medial knee pain that may be seen in OA. The heel wedges used are a quarter of an inch thick along the lateral border and taper medially. Relief was obtained with heel wedges in 74 of 121 knees from 85 patients in one study [46].

Knee orthoses

Common reasons for prescribing orthotics for the knee include:

Pain
Instability caused by ligamentous laxity
Quadriceps weakness
Excess hyperextension of the knee (genu recurvatum) [47–49]

The neoprene sleeve is a commonly prescribed knee brace. It is fabricated with or without holes cut out for the patella. This type of brace may help reduce swelling, provide warmth, and give the patient proprioceptive feedback about the location of the knee in space. Some neoprene sleeves may come with medial and lateral metal bars for added support.

Table 5
Common foot pain etiology and appropriate orthoses for pain relief and preservation of function

Diagnosis	Pain etiology	Orthoses	Function of orthoses
Pes planus (flatfoot)	Hyperpronation at the subtalar joint	University of California Biomechanics Laboratory (UCBL) shoe insert	Symptomatic relief of pain by preventing hyperpronation of the foot
	Ligamentous laxity within the foot	Medial longitudinal arch support	Provides support to arch
Forefoot pain (metatarsalgia)		Metatarsal pad (cookie)–inside shoes	Distributes weight-bearing forces to an area proximal to the metatarsal heads
		Metatarsal bar outside shoe	
Heel pain	Heel spur	Rubber heel pad Calcaneal bar	Reduces pressure on heel
Achilles pain		Heel lift	Decreases stretching forces on Achilles tendon
Plantar fasciitis		Arch support	Decreases stress on medial longitudinal arch during weight-bearing activities
Wide forefoot, cocked toes hallux valgus (seen in rheumatoid arthritis and osteoarthritis)		Wide-toe-box shoes	Relieves pressure on painful deformities of foot
Painful ankle (osteoarthritis)		Rocker bottom shoe	Facilitates movement in a painful ankle [56]
Osteoarthritis medial knee pain		Lateral heel wedges	Unloads medial compartment of knee

A useful brace for quadriceps weakness is the "double metal upright Klenzak" with the ankle positioned in 5° of plantar flexion. This brace hyperextends the knee during the heel-strike phase of the gait cycle and also during stance, which in turn helps stabilize the knee so that it does not buckle when it needs to support the leg [50].

Lenox Hill orthoses may be used to control mediolateral or rotational instability. Hinged orthoses such the Swedish knee cage or Lerhman orthoses may be used to help control sagittal and frontal knee plane motion.

Spinal orthoses

Spinal orthoses are used primarily to relieve pain, limit motion, and support an unstable spine. The soft cervical collars are commonly prescribed orthotics for painful cervical spine conditions. They are believed to work by providing warmth, proprioceptive feedback, and acting as a reminder to the patient to limit motion in painful directions [51].

Hard cervical collars such as Philadelphia, Miami-J, Newport, and Malibu collars offer slightly more support and some limitation of cervical flexion, extension, rotation and lateral bending. A two-poster, four poster, or sterno-occipital mandibular immobilizer collar substantially limits flexion and extension, particularly at C1-C2, but also at C4-C6 [52].

Painful back conditions caused by compression fractures or degenerative disc disease may be relieved by lumbar or thoracic orthoses. These spinal orthotic devices may provide structural support to the spine and reinforce weakened abdominal muscles [53,54].

The lumbosacral (LS) corset is prescribed commonly for patients who have low back pain. Its role is primarily in providing warmth, proprioceptive feedback, and acting as a reminder to limit motion in painful directions. It does not provide structural support or significant restriction of motion of the spine itself. The LS corset is used commonly for short periods of time so that the abdominal and paraspinal musculature does not become atrophied because of disuse. It may be custom molded or come with metal bars on the back.

The thoracolumbosacral orthosis (TLSO) is a hard shell that generally extends from the sacrum to above the inferior angle of the scapulae. It provides significant support to the spine and assists in stabilizing the trunk. It is very confining, however, retains heat, and can be uncomfortable to wear.

There are also thoracic orthoses that limit forward flexion of the thoracic spine. These can be helpful for patients who have compression fractures commonly caused by osteoporosis. Their restricting nature may reduce compliance, however.

Gait aids

Ambulation aids such as canes, crutches, and walkers can be very helpful in reducing pain in the lumbar spine and lower extremities, while maintaining function [55]. They function primarily by unloading the weight placed on painful structures such as the hips, knees, and feet, and improving the base of support for ambulation. Given that there may be an inherent risk in their use, the patient should be trained on the appropriate device by a physical therapist. Muscles of the upper extremities such as the triceps often need to be strengthened, because the arms have the added role of providing support for the lower half of the body.

A cane typically is held by the hand on the nonimpaired part of the body with its upper part at the level of the greater trochanter. The elbow typically is held in 20° of flexion. The role of the cane is to provide the nonimpaired part of the body with extra support as it aids movement of the impaired limb.

Wheelchairs and scooters

The primary function of any assistive device used by the older adult with pain is to reduce pain and maximize function. Wheelchairs (manual and motorized) and scooters can accomplish both.

Wheelchairs can reduce pain by relieving pressure on painful body structures such as the spine and lower extremities. It is always important to check that the patient is prescribed a wheelchair that is appropriate for his/her body dimensions and specific for their impairment(s). Failure to do so may result in pain in the upper extremities (if patient self-propels) or conditions such as pressure ulcers in the sacral spine and greater trochanters.

Scooters are motorized devices that are used commonly by older adults who have painful degenerative conditions of the spine and lower extremities. They require that the operator has intact cognition, good trunk control, and adequate training in its use, and a place to store it.

Summary

Pain negatively impacts quality of life of the older adult in all dimensions, psychologically and physically. By using various pain treatments commonly provided by rehabilitation professionals, physicians caring for the elderly can help their patients to maximize pain control and preserve and/or restore function.

References

[1] National Center for Health Statistic. 1994 second supplement on aging. Available at: www. cdc.gov/nchs/about/otheract/aging/soa2.htm. Accessed January 30, 2006.

[2] Stefen C, Solomon L, Therney-Lesson S, et al. Involvement of medical staff in the assessment of pain. J Pain Symptom Manage 2002;24(3):289–90.

[3] Gaston-Johansson F, Johansson F, Johansson C. Pain in the elderly: prevalence, attitudes, and assessments. Nursing Home Medicine 1996;4:325–31.

[4] Ferrell BA, Ferrell BR, Rivera L. Pain in cognitively impaired nursing home patients. J Pain Symptom Manage 1995;10:591–8.

[5] Wagner AM, Goodwin M, Campbell B, et al. Pain prevalence and pain treatments for residents in Oregon nursing homes. Geriatr Nurs 1997;18:268–72.

[6] Sengstaken EA, King SA. The problems of pain and its detection among geriatric nursing home residents. J Am Geriatr Soc 1993;41:541–4.

[7] Portenoy RK, Lesage P. Management of cancer pain. Lancet 1999;353(9165):1695–700.

[8] CDC. Prevalence of self-reported arthritis or chronic joint symptoms among adults—United States. 2001. MMWR Morbidity and Mortality Weekly Report 2002;51:948–50.

[9] Centers for Disease control and Prevention (CDC). Public health and aging: projected prevalence of self-reported arthritis or chronic joint symptoms among persons aged ≥ 65 years—United States, 2005–2030. MMWR Morb Mortal Wkly Rep 2003;52(21):489–91.

[10] Lawrence RC, Helmick CG, Arnett FC, et al. Estimates of prevalence of arthritis and selected musculoskeletal disorders in the United States. Arthritis Rheum 1998;43: 778–99.

[11] Center for Disease control and Prevention (CDC). Prevalence and impact of arthritis by race and ethnicity—United Stated, 1989–1991. MMWR Morb Mortal Wkly Rep 1996;45:373–8.

[12] Smith HS. Pain taxonomy. In: Pappagallo M, editor. The neurologic basis for pain. New York: McGraw-Hill; 2005. p. 296–7.

[13] Bridges D, Thompson S, Rice AS. Mechanisms of neuropathic pain. Br J Anaesth 2001; 87(1):12–6.

[14] Gallagher RM. Treatment planning in pain medicine. Integrating medical, physical, and behavioral therapies. Med Clin North Am 1999;83:823–49.

[15] Vlaeyen JW, Linton SJ. Fear avoidance and its consequences in chronic musculoskeletal pain: a state of the art. Pain 2000;85:317–32.

[16] Sullivan MJ, Stanish W, Waite H, et al. Catastrophizing pain and disability in patients with soft tissue injuries. Pain 1998;77:253–60.

[17] Keefe FJ, Rumber ME, Scipio CD, et al. Psychological aspects of persistent pain; current state of the science. J Pain 2004;5:195–211.

[18] Stanos SP, Tyburski MD, Harden RN. Management of chronic pain. In: Braddom RL, editor. Physical medicine and rehabilitation. 3rd edition. Elsevier; 2007.

[19] Stanos SP, McLean J, Rader L. Physical medicine rehabilitation approach to pain. Med Clin North Am 2007;91:57–95.

[20] Atchinson JW, Stoll St, Cotter A. Manipulation, traction, and massage. In: Braddom RL, editor. Physical medicine and rehabilitation. 2nd edition. Elsevier; 2007.

[21] Bruce B, Fries JF, Lubeck DP. Aerobic exercise and its impact on musculoskeletal pain in older adults: a 14-ear prospective, longitudinal study. Arthritis Res Ther 2005;7(6): R1263–70.

[22] Taimela S, Diederich C, Hubsch M, et al. The role of physical exercise and inactivity in pain recurrence and absenteeism from work after active outpatient rehabilitation for recurrent or chronic low back pain; a follow-up study. Spine 2000;25(14):1809–16.

[23] Furst G, Gerber L, Smith C. Rehabilitation through learning: energy conservation and joint protection. Baltimore (MD): National Institutes of Health; 1982.

[24] Minor MA, Hewett JE, Webel RS, et al. Efficacy of physical conditioning exercise in patients with rheumatoid arthritis and osteroarthritis. Arthritis Rheum 1989;32:1396–405.

[25] Deschenes M, Kraemer W. Performance and physiologic adaptations to resistance exercise. Am J Phys Med Rehabil 2002;81(Suppl 11):S3–16.

[26] Hart J, Ingersoll C, et al. Weightlifting. In: O'Connor F, Sallis R, Wilder R, editors. Sports medicine: just the facts. New York: McGraw-Hil; 2005. p. 543–7.

[27] Farrell PA, Gates WK, Maksud MG, et al. Increases in plasma beta-endorphin/beta-lipotropin immunoreactivity after treadmill running in humans. J Appl Physiol 1982;52(5):1245–9.

[28] Grossman A, Sutton JR. Endorphins: what are they? How are they measured? What is their role in exercise. Med Sci Sports Exerc 1985;17(1):74–81.

[29] Barrack RL, Skinner H, Cook S, et al. Effect of articulate disease and total knee arthroplasty on knee joint position sense. J Neurophysiol 1983;50(3):684–7.

[30] Barrett DS. Proprioception and function after anterior cruciate reconstruction. J Bone Joint Surg Br 1991;73(5):833–7.

[31] Lichtenstein MJ, Shields SL, Shiavi RG, et al. Clinical determinatis of biomechanics platform measures of balance in aged women. J Am Geriatr Soc 1988;36(11):996–1002.

[32] Lord SR, Sambrook PN, Gilbert C, et al. Postural stability, falls, and fractures in the elderly: results from the Dubbo Osteoporosis Epidemiology Study. Med J Aust 1994;160(11):684–5.

[33] Maki BE, Holliday PJ, Fernie GR. Aging and postural control. A comparison of spontaneous and induced-sway balance tests. J Am Geriatr Soc 1990;38(1):1–9.

[34] Topper AK, Maki BE, Holliday PJ. Are activity-based assessments of balance and gait in the elderly predictive of risk of falling and/or type of fall? J Am Geriatr Soc 1993;41:479–87.

[35] Rozental TD, Sculco TP. Intra-articular corticosteroids: an updated overview. Am J Orthop 2000;29(1):18–23.

[36] Stefanich RJ. Intra-articular corticosteroids in treatment of osteoarthritis. Orthop Rev 1986; 15(2):65–71.

[37] Wobig M, Dickhut A, Maier R, et al. Viscosupplementation with hylan G-F 20: a 26-week controlled trial of efficacy and safety in the osteoarthritic knee. Clin Ther 1998;20(3):410–23.

[38] Kotz R, Kolarz G. Intra-articular hyaluronic acid: duration of effect and results of repeated treatment cycles. Am J Orthop 1999;28(Suppl 11):5–7.

[39] Bellamy N, Campbell J, Robinson V, et al. Viscosupplementation for the treatment of osteoarthritis of the knee. Cochrane Database Syst Rev 2005;2:CD0052321.

[40] Travell JG, Simons DGMyofascial pain and dysfunction, vol. 2. Baltimore (MD): Williams & Wilkins; 1992.

[41] Cummings TM, White AR. Needling therapies in the management of myofascial trigger point pain: a systematic review. Arch Phys Med Rehabil 2001;82:986–92.

[42] Rosen NB. Myofascial pain—the great mimicker and potentiator or muscle pain syndromes. Md Med J 1993;42(3)):261–6.

[43] Redford JB. Orthoses. In: Basmajian JV, Kirby RL, editors. Medical rehabilitation. Baltimore (MD): Williams & Wilkens; 1984. p. 101.

[44] Gerber L, Hunt G. Ankle orthosis for rheumatoid disease. Arthritis Rheum 1985;28:547.

[45] Weist DR, Waters RL, Bontrager EL, et al. The influence of heel design on a rigid ankle foot orthosis. Orthotic and Prosthetic 1979;33:3.

[46] Keating EM, Faris PM, Ritter MA, et al. Use of lateral heel and sole wedges in the treatment of medial osteoarthritis of the knee. Orthop Rev 1993;22:921–4.

[47] Cassuan A, Wunder KE, Fultonberg DM. Orthotic management of the unstable knee. Arch Phys Med Rehabil 1977;58:487–91.

[48] Rubin G, Dixon M, Danisi M. VAPC prescription procedures for knee orthosis and knee-ankle-foot orthosis. Orthotic and Prosthetic 1977;31:9–25.

[49] Smith EM, Juvinoll RC, Corell EB, et al. Bracing the unstable arthritic knee. Arch Phys Med Rebabil 1970;51:22–8.

[50] Sugarbaker PH, Lampert MH. Excision of quadriceps muscle group. Surgery 1983;93: 462–6.

[51] Hartman JT, Palumbo F, Hill BJ. Cineradiography of braced normal cervical spine: comparative study of five commonly used cervical orthoses. Clin Orthop 1975;109:97–102.

[52] Calachis SC Jr, Strohm BS, Ganter EL. Cervical spine motion in normal women: radiographic study of the effect of cervical collars. Arch Phys Med Rebabil 1973;54:161–9.

[53] Bunch WH, Keagy RD. The spine. In: Bunch WH, Keagy RD, editors. Principles of orthotic treatment. St. Louis (MO): CV Mosby; 1976. p. 84–90.

[54] Norton PL, Brown T. The immobilizing efficiency of back braces. Their effect on the posture and motion of the lumbosacral spine. J Bone Joint Surg Am 1957;39:111–39.

[55] Deathe AB, Hayes KC, Winter DA. The biomechanics of canes, crutches, and walkers. Critical Reviews in Physical and Rehabilitation Medicine 1993;5:15–29.

[56] Demopoulous JT. Orthotic and prosthetic management of foot disorders. In: Jahss MH, editor. Disorders of the foot. Philadelphia: WB Saunders; 1982. p. 1785.

ELSEVIER
SAUNDERS

CLINICS IN
GERIATRIC
MEDICINE

Clin Geriatr Med 24 (2008) 335–344

Behavioral Approaches to Pain Management in the Elderly

Lisa J. Norelli, MD, MPH, MRCPsych[a,b,*], Saila K. Harju, MEd[c]

[a]Department of Psychiatry, Albany Medical College, 43 New Scotland Avenue, Albany, NY 12208, USA
[b]Capital District Psychiatric Center, 75 New Scotland Avenue, Albany, NY 12208, USA
[c]Department of Psychology, University of Joensuu, PL11, 80101 Joensuu, Finland

Pain is a common condition and typically undertreated in older adults. It is estimated that chronic pain affects up to half of the elderly living in the community and more than half of those residing in nursing home settings [1–3]. Studies show that older adults are less likely to attend pain management programs and when they do attend are offered fewer treatments [4]. Age-related factors, such as dementia, sensory impairment, pain perception differences, and difficulties expressing pain, are some of the barriers to the assessment and treatment of pain in the elderly [5]. It generally is accepted that pain has a significant negative impact on overall health, functioning, and quality of life. Chronic pain is associated with higher rates of depression, anxiety, cognitive impairment, social isolation, decreased mobility, and sleep disturbances [6,7].

A multidisciplinary and multidimensional approach to the assessment and treatment of pain is recommended for all pain sufferers. Behavioral approaches offer a variety of effective nonpharmacologic treatments for pain management [8,9]. This is a distinct advantage in the older age group. Although analgesics remain the mainstay of treatment for many pain conditions, their use often is limited in the elderly because of higher susceptibility to adverse effects, drug interactions, and increased medical comorbidity. In the broadest sense, behavioral treatments for pain include a diverse range of techniques [10]. This article discusses the evidence for some of the behavioral

* Corresponding author. Department of Psychiatry, Albany Medical College, 43 New Scotland Avenue, Albany, NY 12208.
E-mail address: norelll@mail.amc.edu (L.J. Norelli).

0749-0690/08/$ - see front matter © 2008 Elsevier Inc. All rights reserved.
doi:10.1016/j.cger.2007.12.010   *geriatric.theclinics.com*

approaches commonly available that clinicians can incorporate into to a comprehensive pain management program for older adults. Broadly, these approaches include relaxation methods, hypnosis, behavior therapy, and mind-body conditioning programs.

Relaxation techniques

Relaxation techniques describe a broad group of approaches with diverse origins and methodologies. The common purpose of all these approaches is to achieve a state of physical and mental calmness. Most relaxation techniques share the following characteristics: repetitive focus on something, such as a sound, phrase, body sensation, or muscle tension, and passivity or inattention toward intrusive thoughts and external distractions. Relaxation leads to physiologic changes, such as decreased heart rate and blood pressure. Brief methods include deep breathing and self-control relaxation. Deep relaxation methods, reviewed here, include biofeedback, progressive muscle relaxation (PMR), meditation, and autogenic training. The deep methods are recognized as beneficial in the treatment of chronic pain [11]. Randomized control trials and meta-analyses of the literature support the use of biofeedback and other relaxation therapies in a variety of pain conditions, such as headache, chronic low back pain, and rheumatologic pain [12–15]. There are few studies in the current literature, however, evaluating the use of these techniques specifically in older adults [16].

Biofeedback

Biofeedback typically uses a visual or auditory signal analog of a physiologic measurement to facilitate relaxation training. Over time, individuals learn to control the feedback signal and, therefore, regulate the underlying biologic processes, such as heart rate, blood pressure, and muscle tension. Peripheral skin temperature, galvanic resistance, and electromyography are examples of physiologic measures that commonly are monitored. Biofeedback training often is offered in combination with other treatment interventions in chronic pain rehabilitation programs. Modification of treatment sessions sometimes is necessary to accommodate the elderly, for example, allowing extra time to ensure full understanding of the treatment concepts. Several small studies using biofeedback in older adults have shown significant decreases in pain measures for headache [17–19]. Studies comparing older and younger adults found similar pain reductions with biofeedback in both groups [20].

Progressive muscle relaxation

PMR, developed by Jacobson nearly 100 years ago, is a systematic relaxation method [21]. PMR involves individual tensing and then relaxing of certain muscle groups progressing from one part of the body to the others. With practice, individuals attain the ability to relax quickly using fewer muscle groups until, eventually, they can relax their bodies intentionally without tensing the muscles. PMR can be used alone but frequently is applied in conjunction with other approaches, such as hypnosis and behavior therapies. Greater pain reduction and improved sleep was found in two randomized control studies in older adults enrolled in a wellness program that included PMR, autogenic training, and other relaxation methods compared with usual care [22,23]. Subjects in these studies had a variety of chronic illnesses, including osteoarthritis, rheumatoid arthritis, spinal stenosis, low back pain, and diabetes.

Autogenic training

Autogenic training is a self-directed relaxation technique developed in the early twientieth century by German psychiatrist, Johannes Schultz. With this technique, individuals imagine a relaxing setting and comforting body sensations. This method is practiced for 15 minutes, 3 times daily. There are few reports specific to treating pain in older adults but research in adults suggests there is a role for this method. A 2002 meta-analysis of the clinical effectiveness of autogenic training, completed by Stetter and Kupper [24], found mild to moderate effect size for a range of clinical conditions, including headache, somatoform pain, and Raynaud's disease. A recent trial has shown autogenic training effective in long-term migraine prophylaxis [25].

Meditation

Meditation is guided or self-directed technique for calming the mind and relaxing the body. There are many different meditation approaches, such as mindfulness meditation, concentration meditation, and transcendental meditation. Meditation also is a component of mind-body conditioning techniques, such as tai chi and yoga. Mindfulness meditation allows thoughts, emotions, and sensations to travel through conscious awareness without judgment. Several reviews present clear evidence that mindfulness meditation improves pain and mood and reduces stress [26,27]. Mindfulness meditation is used successfully in older adults who have a range of chronic pain conditions [28,29].

Relaxation techniques have been taught successfully to the elderly to help with a variety of conditions. Some of these methods can be applied in a group format and, once learned, can be self-directed and promote self-efficacy in pain management. These approaches require intact cognitive function, ability to concentration, and regular practice to be effective; therefore, they cannot be used in some older adults who have deficits in these areas.

Hypnosis

Hypnosis is proved an effective analgesic and is at least as effective as other nonpharmacologic techniques, such as cognitive behavior therapy

(CBT), relaxation, and meditation [30]. Simply defined, hypnosis is a state of inner absorption and focused attention often attained through the use of imagery and relaxation techniques. Although in a hypnotic trance, individuals are more receptive to certain communications or suggestions. Through these suggestions, persons can modify their response to pain, including altering their perception of pain and pain-related behaviors. Hypnosis usually is induced by a trained therapist. Some patients can become proficient in the techniques and use self-hypnosis to manage their pain as needed. Hypnosis is known to reduce pain through several mechanisms, including distraction, altering pain perception, rendering it less unpleasant, and increasing the pain threshold by enhancing relaxation and reducing anxiety [31,32]. Some have suggested that older adults are less receptive to hypnosis, but recent studies dispute this notion. Research has found that hypnotizability is a stable trait at least over a 25-year period [33,34]. Research trials of hypnosis and pain often include older adults in the study sample. In their review of controlled trials, Jensen and Patterson [35] confirmed that hypnosis produced significant chronic pain reduction. In some studies, the benefit persisted up to a year after treatment. A recent trial in older adults who had osteoarthitic pain compared the effectiveness of hypnosis, progressive relaxation training, and a control condition. The investigators found that participants in both active treatment groups reported significant decreases in subjective pain with time and used less analgesic medication [36]. For hypnosis to be successful, subjects should have intact cognitive function and ability to concentrate.

Behavior therapies

Behavior therapy approaches to pain management typically are divided into CBT and operant behavior therapy (OBT). Both of these approaches have been used successfully in pain management and pain-related disability. Studies comparing CBT versus OBT in treating chronic low back pain and fibromyalgia found equivalent and clinically significant decreases in pain intensity and physical disability compared with controls [37,38]. A 1999 systematic review and meta-analysis of the literature by Morley and colleagues [39] confirmed that behavior therapy in adults (including CBT, OBT, biofeedback, and relaxation) compared with wait list control conditions, resulted in significant changes in measures of pain experience, mood, cognitive coping and appraisal, pain-related behavior, activity level, and social functioning.

Cognitive behavior therapy

As a form of psychotherapy, CBT focuses on changing individual cognitive activity to subsequently modify associated behaviors, thoughts, and emotions. CBT for pain management is based on a cognitive-behavioral model of pain that states the pain experience is influenced by cognition, affect, and behavior [40]. This principle is taught to patients, with emphasis on their role in controlling their own pain. CBT aims to enhance individual ability to cope with pain effectively through skills training. This often includes relaxation training, such as PMR. The treatment usually is limited to 10 to 12 weekly individual or group sessions. Weekly homework assignments are given to help reinforce key concepts and coping skills [41]. There is compelling evidence that CBT is effective in pain management [42]. For some patients, this treatment restores function, improves mood, and reduces pain and disability. When compared with other active treatments, such as physiotherapy, occupational therapy, and education, CBT demonstrates significantly greater changes in pain experience, cognitive coping and appraisal, and reduced pain-related behavior [39]. There are few studies of CBT in older adults, but recent trials demonstrate the feasibility and efficacy of using CBT to treat pain in the elderly. A pilot study by Reid and colleagues [43] shows CBT effective in reducing pain intensity and pain-related disability in a small sample of cognitively intact older adults who had chronic low back pain.

This approach is not possible for some older adults. CBT requires that participants are cognitively intact, with satisfactory memory and attention, and able to attend weekly treatment sessions and complete homework assignments to reinforce the central strategies learned in the treatment sessions.

Operant behavior therapy

OBT is based on the principles of operant conditioning, that is, the use of consequences to modify the behaviors. Consequences frequently include positive and negative reinforcements. In this context, OBT interventions are aimed at reducing learned pain-related behaviors and the degree to which pain interferes with daily functioning. Learned pain behaviors often interfere with recovery and can be encouraged and reinforced in sufferers by family or society. For example, when in pain, individuals are absolved of unpleasant responsibilities and receive extra sympathy or attention from loved ones [44]. These rewarding responses to being in pain can reinforce the sick role. Behaviors compatible with wellness tend to be extinguished, and passive activities (eg, not exerting oneself or watching television) are encouraged. OBT involves interventions, such as increasing physical activity, physiotherapy, analgesic management, and inclusion of significant others, to reduce the reinforcement of learned pain behavior and increase reward for wellness behavior. OBT has been applied successfully to a variety of chronic pain conditions; however, there is a paucity of data regarding the use of OBT for pain management specifically in older adults [5,45,46].

Despite the lack of research, it is expected that behavior therapy approaches can be applied successfully across the lifespan. Where appropriate, clinicians typically combine aspects of supportive, behavioral, and cognitive therapy approaches when working with older individuals who have pain.

Mind-body conditioning practices

Beyond physiotherapy and exercise, other movement-based methods hold promise in the management of pain conditions in older adults. These approaches include physical and mental conditioning systems, such as yoga, tai chi, and qigong. Mind-body conditioning routines have been in use for thousands of years and increasingly adopted by Western society as part of healthy lifestyle regimes. These systems are practiced for their beneficial effects on the body and mind and also applied for therapeutic effects. Generally these conditioning routines are low impact. They can be applied individually or in groups and easily tailored to different physical limitations and treatment settings; therefore, they are suited for some older adults ideally.

Tai chi and qigong are different systems but both entail practicing a series of routines including slow, controlled movements, mental concentration, and focused breathing believed to enhance the body's energy (chi or qi) and facilitate its healthy flow [47]. Yoga typically involves using a series of postures and movements, meditation, and breathing exercises to achieve higher physical, mental, and spiritual development. Potential health benefits include increased physical strength, flexibility, mental calmness, and focus. Positive general health effects for all adult age groups are supported by clinical research findings. In healthy older adults, tai chi is shown to improve perceived physical function, hypertension, balance, and risk for falls [48]. In a group of frail older adults, tai chi enhanced a variety of measures, including body mass index, heart rate, and systolic blood pressure [49,50]. Qigong therapy is demonstrated to enhance mood and hormonal and immunologic function in healthy male adults compared with controls [51]. In a group of cardiac rehabilitation patients, those who participated in qigong had improved perceived physical activity level, balance, and coordination as compared with controls [52]. Studies on the use of yoga in older adults demonstrate lower blood pressure and enhanced general psychologic well-being, quality of life, and physical function [53–55].

There are few studies examining the use of yoga, tai chi, and qigong specifically for the treatment of pain in older adults. Two research trials using yoga to treat osteoarthritis in older adults found significant improvements in pain measures and physical function [56,57]. Similarly, several controlled trials of yoga for chronic low back pain in older adults demonstrated significant improvement in pain and function [58–60]. These benefits persisted at a 3-month follow up assessment [59]. A small study in community-residing older adults who had arthritis demonstrated significant improvement in health satisfaction and self-efficacy of those attending tai chi classes as compared with controls [61,62]. Another study in which older women who had osteoarthritis were randomized to tai chi or a telephone contact control group showed significant improvement in joint pain, stiffness, and physical function [63]. In a general health study that looked at pain as one outcome measure, qigong improved body pain and lowered blood pressure and heart rates [64]. Additional studies of qigong as an intervention for the elderly who had chronic pain found significant improvements in mood and pain measures [65,66].

The research on different mind-body conditioning programs is limited but does support the feasibility and the safety of these therapies. Evidence suggests a potential role in the treatment of pain in older adults. Although further research is needed in this area, it is conceivable that many of these movement principles could be adapted to the elderly population, even those who have significant cognitive and physical disabilities.

Summary

Pain is a complex phenomenon, influenced by many individual and external factors, and may be experienced differently with age. The detrimental health and social effects of chronic pain are well known. Age-related disorders, such as dementia, may interfere with the communication of pain. Health care provider bias and cultural expectations also may be barriers to the recognition and management of pain in the elderly. A multidisciplinary and multimodal approach in older adults is essential to effective assessment and management. Behavioral approaches to pain should be considered and incorporated into treatment where appropriate. Behavioral treatments are feasible, effective, and generally carry low risk. These methods also have other desired effects aside from pain relief. Additional health benefits include improvement in mood, anxiety, functioning, and quality of life and decreased need for analgesic medication.

There are limitations in the use of some of these approaches in patients who have significant cognitive impairment or physical limitations. For example, memory, attention, and concentration are requisites for participation in hypnosis, CBT, and some relaxation methodologies. The core principles of relaxation, movement or conditioning techniques, and behavior-modifying responses, however, can be adapted to individualized pain management programs. The movement-based modalities, such as tai chi, may be more adaptable to accommodate those individuals who have significant cognitive deficits. Despite the scarcity of clinical trials in the use of these techniques in the elderly, there is considerable evidence for their effectiveness in some patient groups, especially in combination with pharmacologic therapy. Future research in this area should focus on studying these approaches separately and in combination, particularly in older adults in a variety of settings.

References

[1] Ferrell BA, Ferrell BR, Osterweil D. Pain in the nursing home. J Am Geriatr Soc 1990;38: 409–14.
[2] Helme RD, Gibson SJ. The epidemiology of pain in elderly people. Clin Geriatr Med 2001; 17:417–31.

[3] Mobily PR, Herr KA, Clark MK, et al. An epidemiologic analysis of pain in the elderly: the Iowa 65+ rural health study. J Aging Health 1994;6:139–45.

[4] Kee WG, Middlaugh SJ, Redpath S, et al. Age as a factor in admission to chronic pain rehabilitation. Clin J Pain 1998;14:121–8.

[5] Helme RD. Chronic pain management in older people. Eur J Pain 2001;5:31–6.

[6] Bair MJ, Robinson RL, Katon W, et al. Depression and pain comorbidity: a literature review. Arch Intern Med 2003;163:2433–45.

[7] Ettinger WH Jr, Fried LP, Harris T, et al. Self-reported causes of physical disability in older people: the Cardiovascular Health Study. CHS Collaborative Research Group. J Am Geriatr Soc 1994;42:1035–44.

[8] Cavalieri TA. Pain management in the elderly. J Am Osteopath Assoc 2002;102:481–5.

[9] Gibson SJ. IASP global year against pain in older persons: highlighting the current status and future perspectives in geriatric pain. Expert Rev Neurother 2007;7:627–35.

[10] Morone NE, Greco CM. Mind-body interventions for chronic pain in older adults: a structured review. Pain Med 2007;8:359–75.

[11] Integration of behavioral and relaxation approaches into the treatment of chronic pain and insomnia. NIH Technol Statement. 1995;1–34 [online]. Available at: http://consensus.nih.gov/1995/1995BehaviorRelaxPainInsomnia017html.htm. Accessed August 1, 2007.

[12] Astin JA. Mind-body therapies for the management of pain. Clin J Pain 2004;20:27–32.

[13] Flor H, Birbaumer N. Comparison of the efficacy of electromyographic biofeedback, cognitive-behavior therapy, and conservative medical interventions in the treatment of chronic musculoskeletal pain. J Consult Clin Psychol 1993;61:653–8.

[14] Holroyd KA, Penzien DB. Client variables and the behavioral treatment of recurrent tension headache: a meta-analytic review. J Behav Med 1986;9:515–36.

[15] Malone MD, Strube MJ, Scogin FR. Meta-analysis of non-medical treatments for chronic pain. Pain 1988;34:231–44.

[16] Arena JG, Hightower NE, Chong GC. Relaxation therapy for tension headache in the elderly. A prospective study. Psychol Aging 1988;3:96–8.

[17] Arena JG, Hannah SL, Bruno GM, et al. Electromyographic biofeedback training for tension headache in the elderly: a prospective study. Biofeedback Self Regul 1991;16:379–90.

[18] Kabela E, Blanchard EB, Appelbaum KA, et al. Self-regulatory treatment of headache in the elderly. Biofeedback Self Regul 1989;14:219–28.

[19] Nicholson NL, Blanchard EB. A controlled evaluation of behavioral treatment of chronic headache in the elderly. Behav Ther 1993;24:395–408.

[20] Middaugh SJ, Pawlick K. Biofeedback and behavioral treatment of persistent pain in the older adult: a review and study. Appl Psychophysiol Biofeedback 2002;27:185–202.

[21] Jacobson E. Progressive relaxation. A physiological and clinical investigation of muscular states and their significance in psychology and medical practice. Chicago: University of Chicago Press; 1974.

[22] Rybarczyk B, Demarco G, Delacruz M, et al. A classroom mind/body wellness intervention for older adults with chronic illness: comparing immediate and 1 year benefits. Behav Med 2001;27:15–27.

[23] Rybarczyk B, Demarco G, Delacruz M, et al. Comparing mind-body wellness interventions for older adults with chronic illness: classroom vs home instruction. Behav Med 1999;24:181–90.

[24] Stetter F, Kupper S. Autogenic training: a meta-analysis of clinical outcome studies. Appl Psychophysiol Biofeedback 2002;27:45–98.

[25] Juhasz G, Zsombok T, Gonda X, et al. Effects of autogenic training on nitroglycerin-induced headaches. Headache 2007;47:371–83.

[26] Baer RA. Mindfulness training as a clinical intervention: a conceptual and empirical review. Clinical Psychology Science and Practice 2003;10:125–43.

[27] Grossman P, Niemann L, Schmidt S, et al. Mindfulness-based stress reduction and health benefits: a meta-analysis. J Psychosom Res 2004;57:35–43.

[28] Morone NE, Greco CM, Weiner DK. Mindfulness meditation for the treatment of chronic low back pain in older adults: a randomized controlled pilot study. Pain 2008;134:310–9.

[29] Kabat-Zinn J. An outpatient program in behavioral medicine for chronic pain patients based on the practice of mindfulness meditation: theoretical considerations and preliminary results. Gen Hosp Psychiatry 1982;4:33–47.

[30] Montgomery GH, DuHamel KN, Redd WH. A meta-analysis of hypnotically induced analgesia: how effective is hypnosis? Int J Clin Exp Hypn 2000;48:138–53.

[31] Patterson DR, Jensen MP. Hypnosis and clinical pain. Psychol Bull 2003;129:495–521.

[32] Holroyd J. Hypnosis treatment of clinical pain: understanding why hypnosis is useful. Int J Clin Exp Hypn 1996;44:33–51.

[33] Morgan AH, Hilgard ER. Age differences in susceptibility to hypnosis. Int J Clin Exp Hypn 1973;21:78–85.

[34] Piccione C, Hilgard ER, Zimbardo P. On the degree of stability of measured hypnotizability over a 25 year period. J Pers Soc Psychol 1989;56:289–95.

[35] Jensen M, Patterson DR. Hypnotic treatment of chronic pain. J Behav Med 2006;29:95–124.

[36] Gay MC, Philippot P, Luminet O. Differential effectiveness of psychological interventions for reducing osteoarthritis pain: a comparison of Erikson hypnosis and Jacobson relaxation. Eur J Pain 2002;6:1–16.

[37] Thieme K, Turk DC, Flor H. Responder criteria for operant and cognitive-behavioral treatment for fibromyalgia syndrome. Arthritis Rheum 2007;15:830–6.

[38] Nicholas MK, Wilson PH, Goyen J. Operant-behavioral and cognitive-behavioral treatment for low back pain. Behav Res Ther 1991;29:225–38.

[39] Morley S, Eccleston C, Williams A. Systematic review and meta-analysis of randomized controlled trials of cognitive behavioral therapy for chronic pain in adults, excluding headache. Pain 1999;80:1–13.

[40] Turk DC, Meichenbaum D, Genest M. Pain and behavioral medicine: a cognitive-behavioral perspective. New York: Guilford Press; 1983.

[41] Keefe FJ. Cognitive therapy for managing pain. Clin Psychol 1996;49:4–5.

[42] Kerns RD, Otis JD, Marcus KS. Cognitive-behavior therapy for chronic pain in the elderly. Clin Geriatr Med 2001;17:503–23.

[43] Reid MC, Otis J, Barry LC, et al. Cognitive-behavioral therapy for chronic low back pain in older persons: a preliminary study. Pain Med 2003;4:223–30.

[44] Tyrer SP. Learned pain behavior. BMJ 1986;292:1–2.

[45] Thieme K, Gromnica-Ihle E, Flor H. Operant behavioral treatment of fibromyalgia: a controlled study. Arthritis Rheum 2003;49:314–20.

[46] Vlaeyen JWS, Haazen IWCJ, Schuerman JA, et al. Behavioral rehabilitation of chronic low back pain: comparison of an operant treatment, an opernt cognitive treatment, and an operant respondent treatment. Br J Clin Psychol 1995;43:95–118.

[47] Sancier KM. Medical applications of qigong and emitted qi on humans, animals, cell cultures, and plants: a review of selected scientific research. Am J Acupunct 1991;19:367–77.

[48] Young DR, Appel LJ, Jee S, et al. The effects of aerobic exercise and t'ai chi on blood pressure in older people: results of a randomized trial. J Am Geriatr Soc 1999;47:277–84.

[49] Wolf SL, Barnhart HX, Kutner NG, et al. Reducing frailty and falls in the older persons: an investigation of tai chi and computerized balance training. J Am Geriatr Soc 2003;51:1794–803.

[50] Wolf SL, O'Grady M, Easley KA, et al. The influence of intense tai chi training on physical performance and hemodynamic outcomes in transitionally frail, older adults. J Gerontol A Biol Sci Med Sci 2006;61:184–9.

[51] Lee MS, Huh HJ, Hong SS, et al. Psychoneuroimmunological effects of Qi-therapy: preliminary study on the changes of level of anxiety, mood, cortisol and melatonin and cellular function of neutrophil and natural killer cells. Stress and Health 2001;17:17–24.

[52] Stenlund T, Lindstrom B, Granlund M, et al. Cardiac rehabilitation for the elderly: Qi gong and group discussions. Eur J Cardiovasc Prev Rehabil 2005;12:5–11.

[53] Haber D. Yoga as a preventive health care program for white and black elders: an exploratory study. Int J Aging Hum Dev 1983;17:169–76.

[54] Oken BS, Zajdel D, Kishiyama S, et al. Randomized, controlled, six-month trial of yoga in healthy seniors: effects on cognition and quality of life. Altern Ther Health Med 2006;12: 40–7.

[55] Dibenedetto M, Innes KE, Taylor AG, et al. Effect of a gentler Iyengar yoga program on gait in the elderly: an exploratory study. Arch Phys Med Rehabil 2005;86:1830–7.

[56] Kolasinski SL, Garfinkel M, Tsai AG, et al. Iyengar yoga for treating symptoms of osteoarthritis of the knees: a pilot study. J Altern Complement Med 2005;11:689–93.

[57] Garfinkel MS, Schumacher HR Jr, Hussain A, et al. Evaluation of yoga based regimen for treatment of osteoarthritis of the hands. J Rheumatol 1994;21:2341–3.

[58] Sherman KJ, Cherkin DC, Erro J, et al. Comparing yoga, exercise, and a self-care book for chronic low back pain: a randomized, controlled trial. Ann Intern Med 2005;143:849–56.

[59] Williams KA, Petronis J, Smith D, et al. Effect of Iyengar yoga therapy for chronic low back pain. Pain 2005;115:107–17.

[60] Galantino ML, Bzdewka TM, Eissler-Russo JL, et al. The impact of modified Hatha yoga on chronic low back pain: a pilot study. Altern Ther Health Med 2004;10:56–9.

[61] Hartman CA, Manos TM, Winter C, et al. Effects of t'ai chi training on function and quality of life indicators in older adults with osteoarthritis. J Am Geriatr Soc 2000;48:1553–9.

[62] Li F, Harmer P, Mcauley E, et al. Tai chi, self-efficacy, and physical function in the elderly. Prev Sci 2001;2:229–39.

[63] Song R, Lee EO, Lam P, et al. Effects of tai chi exercise on pain, balance, muscle strength, and perceived difficulties in physical functioning in older women with osteoarthritis: a randomized clinical trial. J Rheumatol 2003;30:2039–44.

[64] Cheung BM, Lo JL, Fong DY, et al. Randomized controlled trial of qigong in the treatment of mild essential hypertension. J Hum Hypertens 2005;19:697–704.

[65] Lee MS, Yang KH, Huh HJ, et al. Qi therapy as an intervention to reduce chronic pain and to enhance mood in elderly subjects: a pilot study. Am J Chin Med 2001;29:237–45.

[66] Yang KH, Kim YH, Lee MS. Efficacy of Qi-therapy (external Qigong) for elderly people with chronic pain. Int J Neurosci 2005;115:949–63.

CLINICS IN
GERIATRIC
MEDICINE

Clin Geriatr Med 24 (2008) 345–368

Interventional Techniques for Back Pain

William F. Lavelle, MD[a],*,
Elizabeth Demers Lavelle, MD[b],
Howard S. Smith, MD[c]

[a]Department of Orthopaedic Surgery, The Cleveland Clinic Foundation, Cleveland Clinic
Center for Spine Health, 9500 Euclid Avenue, Desk A41, Cleveland, OH 44195, USA
[b]The Cleveland Clinic Foundation Department of Anesthesiology, Cleveland Clinic,
9500 Euclid Avenue, Cleveland, OH 44195, USA
[c]Department of Anesthesiology, Albany Medical Center, 47 New Scotland Avenue,
MC-131, Albany, NY 12208, USA

Most of the United States population will be afflicted by some form of spine related pain, with the common cold as the only more common source of missed days of work [1,2]. Typically, patients in their third to fifth decade of their life will experience either low back pain or some form of sciatica. Older patients also experience back pain, with the most frequent causes being lumbar spinal stenosis or vertebral compression fractures. Fortunately, most back pain is self-limited; however, a subset of these patients will need interventional techniques in their care [3]. Minimally invasive interventional techniques in the treatment of back pain, lumbosacral radicular pain, lumbar spinal stenosis, and compression fractures are reviewed.

Minimally invasive techniques for the treatment of axial back pain

The human spine is a complex and dynamic structure that intricately but not flawlessly combines support with motion. Posteriorly, there are four facet joints associated with each vertebra, while the vertebral bodies themselves are separated by intervertebral discs. Mechanical failure of any of these motion segments may cause or contribute to back pain. Pain may be generated from any number of the intricate structures in and around the spine. It is the challenge of the physician to determine the source of the pain and provide treatment.

---

* Corresponding author.
E-mail address: lavellwf@yahoo.com (W.F. Lavelle).

The truly savvy patient will seek a name for his or her affliction. Unfortunately, of patients who present to a primary care physician, most will leave their doctor's office without a definitive diagnosis. Less than 10% of patients will have an identifiable cause for their back pain such as a fracture, spondylolisthesis, or a tumor [4,5]. Most of this nonspecific back pain is attributable to normal aging and degeneration.

The human spine often fails in a predictable pattern. The disc appears to be afflicted first. The biochemical environment of the intervertebral disc changes remarkably, as people age. The disc loses its water and alters its chemical content, with the overall content of proteoglycan, collagen, and water decreasing. Proteoglycans and water allow the disc to resist compression, while collagen provides structure and maintains disc integrity. These changes cause aged discs to have decreased stiffness and strength. Disc failure is merely the beginning of a series of failures in the spine [6,7]. Failure of the disc is followed soon by hypertrophy and failure of the supporting ligaments, followed by the facet joints [8,9].

Pain is often a direct result of inflammation. This inflammation may be a result of direct injury or motion. Increased motion caused by disk degeneration, combined with decreased shear resistance, may allow for an anterior translation of the vertebral body, resulting in a condition termed spondylolisthesis. Spondylolisthesis may be unstable and therefore painful. Spondylolisthesis has been classified with multiple schemes, but general categories include: dysplastic/developmental, traumatic (acute, chronic), degenerative, and pathologic.

Back pain also may be caused by isolated changes in the internal disc environment. Internal disc derangement (IDD) is a term coined by Crock in 1970 [10]. The term IDD was made to describe a large group of patients whose disabling back and leg pain worsened after an operation for suspected disc prolapse. IDD was intended to describe a condition marked by an alteration in the internal structure and metabolic functions of disc that were felt to be attributable to one particular injury or a series of injuries that may have even been subclinical. The annulus and the vertebral endplates possess nerve fibers that may be irritated by IDD. Tears in the annulus fibrosus are felt to be either the major manifestation of IDD or a contributor of IDD pain [10–12].

Discography

Needle puncture of the intervertebral disc first was performed in Scandinavia by Lindgren in 1941 [13,14]. In 1948, Hirsch [13] was the first to use this technique to aide in the diagnosis of painful discs. Lindblom [15] made the addition of injecting contrast material to help visualize annular tears. Disc disruptions, which allow the nerve endings located in the annulus to be exposed to the inflammatory molecules produced by nuclear degradation, are felt to be a possible cause of painful discs. The primary diagnostic element of a discogram remains the provocation of the patient's usual pain upon injection of the ailing disc, while contrast injection provides additional information about the character of the disc in question.

As discography is merely a tool to aide in a clinical diagnosis, a thorough understanding of a patient's pain is necessary. As with all diagnostic aides, results must be framed in the proper context of additional patient information. A pain diagram may be a useful addition to the clinical history before performing a discogram [14].

Discography may be performed in various patient positions. The choice of positioning often is based on physician preference. The most common patient positions are prone and lateral. If numerous percutaneous procedures are planned, then it is best to place a patient in a position that is comfortable. This will decrease patient movement facilitating the procedure. Positioning also should be considered when trying to visualize difficult structures. Oblique positioning, particularly positioning the patient at a 45° angle, allows for better visualization of the lumbosacral junction [16].

Patients often prefer mild procedural sedation such as midazolam; however, the primary endpoint of discography is the provocation of pain. Patient interaction during the procedure is a necessity. Modern fluoroscopic guidance has allowed for accurate needle positioning. Discography of the upper lumbar spine (L3–4 and L2–3) typically is performed with a simple anteroposterior and lateral view to align the fluoroscope with the endplates of the disc level in question. After localization, the fluoroscope tower is turned to an oblique angle until the anterior aspect of the superior facet joint is positioned at a point where 40% of the disk is anterior and 60% is posterior. Once fluoroscope positioning is adequate, the skin is prepared surgically and infiltrated with a small amount of a local anesthetic. Under live fluoroscopic guidance, the needle is passed as close to the anterior aspect of the superior articular process of the facet as possible. The needle must pass between the superior articular process and the exiting nerve root (Fig. 1). Shooting leg pain suggests contact with the nerve root. Resistance will be encountered upon entering the disc. At the conclusion of needle placement, the needle should be at the center of the disc in all fluoroscopic projections. Lower lumbar levels are more difficult to approach because of the presence of the iliac crests. Visualization of the lumbosacral junction typically requires a cranial tilt of the C-arm to 45°.

All levels to be investigated should have 22-gauge spinal needles placed. Typically, at least one control level also should be selected in addition to the levels being investigated. Once all needles are positioned, a water-based contrast agent such as a low osmolar, nonionic, iodinated contrast is injected into each level being tested. A standard injection worksheet is recommended to help standardize the injections. Typically, a worksheet should include: the volume of contrast injected, the character of the pain, whether the pain provoked by the discogram mirrors the patient's typical pain, the amount of

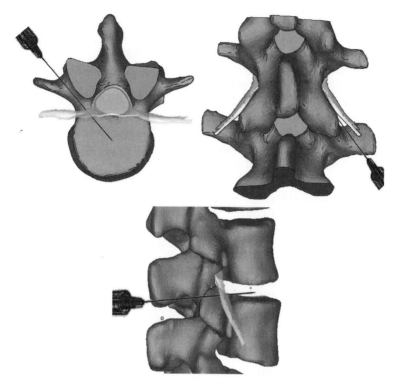

Fig. 1. Disc injection positioning. For proper intradiscal placement, the needle is passed between the superior articular process and the exiting nerve root.

contrast-induced pressure the disc can maintain, and the integrity of the disc. Internal disc derangement findings include:

- CT discography reveals an annular tear.
- Pain should be reproduced on a discogram.
- As a control, stimulation of at least one other disc should fail to reproduce pain.

An incompetent disc rapidly leak contrast will and be unable to hold a significant amount of contrast pressure. The specificity of discography may be improved if a positive disc is defined as one in which:

- Evoked concordant or similar/familiar pain-numerical rating scale of at least 6 at a pressure above opening pressure of no more than 50 psi and total volume injected no more than 3 mL
- The morphology is abnormal–high-grade annual disruption (grade 3 or higher)

Although rare, complications have been reported because of discography. These include neural injury, bleeding, and intradural leakage of the injected material [16]. Infection is often the most significant risk associated with discography, with a rate of postdiscography discitis reported as up to 1.3% per disc [16–18].

The usefulness of discography remains debated. When combined with MRI, some studies have found that patients who had discography-induced concordant pain and an MRI-documented abnormality fared well 75% of the time with single-level L5–S1 fusion. Patients in whom MRI revealed normal findings but in whom discography provoked concordant pain only had a favorable outcome 50% of the time [19]. A recent systematic review of the literature was published that assessed the diagnostic accuracy of discography with respect to chronic spinal pain. The study found strong evidence of the diagnostic accuracy of discography as an imaging tool. It found strong evidence of the ability of discography to evoke pain. There was strong evidence supporting the role of discography in identifying that subset of patients who had lumbar discogenic pain. The review found moderate evidence supporting the role of discography in identifying a subset of patients who had cervical discogenic pain. There was limited evidence supporting the role of discography in identifying a subset of patients who had thoracic discogenic pain [20]. They concluded that overall, discography was a useful imaging and pain evaluation tool for identifying a subset of patients who have chronic spinal pain secondary to intervertebral disc disorders.

Intradiscal electrothermal therapy

Percutaneous intradiscal electrothermal therapy (IDET) is a new treatment that has been developed for patients with imaging and discographic evidence of internal disc disruption (IDD) that was approved by the US Food and Drug Administration (FDA) in 1998. This minimally invasive technique uses a navigable catheter to provide targeted thermal energy within the disc. The catheter is placed in an identical manner as a needle used for a discogram. This procedure has the advantage of preserving the native disc structure. The procedure is dependent on the premise of thermocoagulation of nociceptors in the annulus [21,22]. Once in the disc space, the catheter heats the disc to a temperature of 90°C over the course of 15 to 20 minutes [23]. Undergoing the IDET procedure does not eliminate the possibility for surgery at a later time. Although the literature on this new technique is limited, studies have found that between 50% and 65% of patients reported a significant reduction in their back pain after an IDET procedure. A recent meta-analysis found a statistically significant decrease in pain after treatment. The authors found a mean improvement of 2.9 points on the visual analog scale and a mean improvement of 21 points on the back pain subscale of the Medical Outcomes Study 36-item Short-Form Health Survey (SF-36) [24]. A similar review concluded the opposite. This review was based on fewer but higher-quality randomized control trials. The authors found that there is little support for the efficacy or effectiveness of percutaneous thermocoagulation intradiscal techniques for treating discogenic low back pain [25].

Facet injections

Patients who have primarily facet degeneration rather than significant disc disease often complain of greater discomfort with spine extension or hyperextension positioning. Further degeneration may allow any position to provoke pain. As a minimally invasive diagnostic and therapeutic modality, facet joint injections may be offered.

Not all physicians support the use of facet injections, with some doubting their clinical efficacy entirely. There are only a few well-performed and controlled studies examining the efficacy of facet injections. Mild symptomatic improvement has been touted by numerous investigations; however, there are just as many studies reporting limited if any improvement in back pain as the result of facet injections.

As with many local blocks, facet injections originally were performed with large volumes of anesthetic and steroid. The facet joints themselves were localized by palpation. Modern techniques use imaging techniques for facet localization. Facet block techniques using CT have been described; however, most physicians use fluoroscopy. This is likely because fluoroscopic guidance is widely available and imparts a lower radiation load to the patient and the physician. The desired facet joint is localized on orthogonal images. The needle is introduced into the skin and advanced incrementally into the facet joint under live fluoroscopy. The physician placing the block may choose to use radioprotective gloves or a surgical instrument such as a needle driver in an attempt to minimize direct radiation exposure to the physician's hands. Most physicians describe a pop upon entering the facet joint capsule, although this response may be diminished in the arthritic facet joint (Fig. 2).

Contrast material may be injected to confirm proper needle placement. The needle may deflect noticeably upon entering the facet joint. Some physicians feel the injection needle should be placed near the notch between the transverse process and the superior articulating process, as this is the site where the sensory nerve branches enter the bone. The usefulness of this

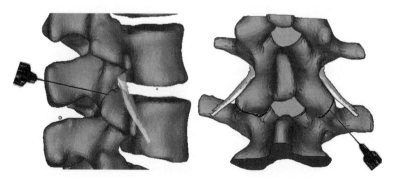

Fig. 2. Positioning for facet injection. The needle is guided fluoroscopically into the facet joint. A pop has been described but may be diminished in the truly diseased facet.

technique also is debated, as it does not allow for any direct introduction of medication into the facet joint. This technique of medial branch nerve block, however, may be used in attempts to prolong efficacy with radiofrequency denervation.

Once the proper positioning has been confirmed, a mixture of steroid and local anesthetic is injected. The choice of steroid is primarily physician preference. Many clinicians prefer to use steroid solutions of relatively small particle size (eg, Soluspan [Celestone]) out of the belief that they are safer if injected into the spinal cord vasculature accidentally. Classically, the duration of a steroid's effect should be inversely proportional to solubility of the steroid. Unfortunately, there are few studies that address the clinical superiority of one agent over another. Clinicians typically choose medical agents based on familiarity. Patients often report immediate relief, but may report transient worsening of symptoms. This may be because of capsular distention or a steroid flair reaction.

A recent review found some support for the use of facet injections. The review encompassed randomized and nonrandomized trials using the criteria established by the Agency for Healthcare Research and Quality (AHRQ) [26]. The review found that for lumbar intra-articular facet joint injections, there was moderate evidence for short- and long-term improvement. The evidence was limited for cervical intra-articular facet joint injections for short- and long-term pain relief. For cervical, thoracic, and lumbar medial branch blocks with local anesthetics (with or without steroids), the evidence supporting efficacy was moderate for short- and long-term pain relief with repeat injections. The evidence for pain relief with radiofrequency neurotomy of cervical and lumbar medial branch nerves is moderate for short- and long-term pain relief, and indeterminate for thoracic facet neurotomy [26]. Although this review concluded an overall positive effect for facet injections, this fact remains ardently debated in the spine community.

Open surgery for painful motion segments

Most painful joints in the body ultimately may be treated either by arthroplasty or fusion. The spine is no different. Despite the recent popularity of disc arthroplasty, fusion remains the standard of care for painful motion segments that have failed conservative treatment.

Fusion techniques are designed to selectively address the painful motion segments. The posterior facet joints, the anterior disc, or a combined approach where both the anterior and posterior motion segments are fused may be used. As with most fusion procedures used in orthopedic surgery, the fusion process should excise or denude the joint that has been painful completely. Paramount to durability and functionality of the fusion is for the procedure to restore the patient to an anatomic and functional position so as to lessen the stress on the adjacent joints that may be prone to future degeneration [27].

Minimally invasive techniques for treating lumbar disc disease

The condition of spine-related pain or paresthesia that radiates into the legs and/or buttocks has been referred to by various names including: the general term—sciatica, or more precise terms if the symptoms are dermatomal or myotomal—lumbosacral radicular pain, lumbosacral radiculalgia. Lumbosacral radicular pain may be attributed to numerous causes, including herniated discs, congenital stenosis, hypertrophied facets, and/or hypertrophied ligaments. All of these entities have the common factor of extrinsic nerve compression. Some physicians and basic scientists feel that lumbosacral radicular pain cannot be explained entirely by a pressure phenomenon [28,29]. As stated earlier, the intervertebral disc themselves contain proinflammatory molecules that have been found to excite nerve roots [30].

Disc failure

Throughout life, discs see tremendous forces imparted by cyclic loading that causes mechanical destruction. This destruction is felt to only be a component of the entire degenerative cascade. The mechanical destruction is accompanied by a cascade of nonreversible cell-mediated responses causing cell death or apoptosis. Cadaveric experiments and computer models have shown how various combinations of compression, bending, and torsion can cause the morphologic features of disc degeneration such as endplate disruption, fissure formation in the annulus, radial bulging, disc prolapses, and internal collapse of the annulus [31]. As the annulus eventually fails, typically through a small rent or fracture, the nucleus pulposus material is pushed slowly through the annular ring of the disc. Current understanding of the process of disc failure is limited; therefore, the ability to mitigate the damage caused by degenerative processes also is limited. Studies have shown that with time, the number of blood vessels in the vertebral end plates decreases, with most disappearing by the time a patient is 30. The chemical structure of the disc and organization of the disc change with age [32]. Collagen fibril organization is altered, with its absolute concentration decreasing with age. The amount of proteoglycans also declines as discs age, with the ratio of keratin to chondroitin sulfate changing. Little is known about the implications of these changes; however, these alterations theoretically would diminish the disc's ability to withstand compressive forces.

The American Society of Interventional Pain Physicians publishes guidelines for interventional techniques in the management of chronic spinal pain every 2 years [33].

Epidural steroid injections

Epidural steroid injections (ESIs) are a commonly used minimally invasive treatment for low back pain and lumbosacral radicular pain. The first epidural injection was performed in 1901 with a caudal approach using cocaine to treat sciatica and lumbago. Epidural steroids first were introduced into the epidural space to treat lumbar radicular pain in 1952 by Robecci. Since that time, further investigations have been performed demonstrating the clinical improvement of pain symptoms in patients who have ESIs [34].

The success of epidural steroids is based on the fact that inflammation at the epidural space and nerve roots secondary to mechanical compression from a herniated disc or other mechanism is a significant factor in the cause of radicular pain [35,36]. Because lumbar radicular pain may originate from inflammation of epidural space and the nerve root, analgesic effects of corticosteroids may be related to the inhibition of phospholipase A2 with decreased resultant inflammation, inhibition of neural transmission in nociceptive C-fibers, and the reduction of capillary permeability.

Lumbar epidural steroid injection procedure

Patients who have low back pain, radiculopathy, or neurogenic claudication may be potential candidates for an ESI. Available imaging on the patient, including plain films and MRI images should be reviewed, although there is not always a direct relationship between a patient's MRI and the true cause of his or her pain. The contraindications for an ESI are listed in Box 1.

Epidural steroid injections may be performed in the cervical, thoracic, or lumbar regions by means of translaminar or transforaminal approaches. The translaminar, also referred to as the interlaminar approach, may be done paramedian or midline. With the translaminar approach, the epidural needle enters the skin, then the subcutaneous tissue—the paraspinal muscles in the paramedian approach or the interspinous ligament in the midline approach—and finally the ligamentum flavum (Fig. 3). With the transforaminal approach, the epidural needle is placed in the neuroforamen ventral to the nerve root, then directed obliquely until the tip of the needle touches the

---

Box 1. Contraindications to epidural steroid injections

Absolute contraindications
Uncontrolled bleeding /anticoagulation
Local cellulitis near injection site
Systemic infection
Uncontrolled diabetes mellitus
Progressive neurologic disorder
Cauda equina syndrome

Relative contraindications
History of laminectomy at proposed level of injection
Allergy to contrast media
Allergy to local anesthetic

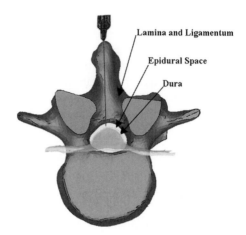

Lamina and Ligamentum

Epidural Space

Dura

Fig. 3. Lumbar epidural steroid injection. The needle is positioned between the lamina/ligamentum and the dura.

posterior lateral portion of the vertebral body, just under the pedicle. The caudal approach also may be used for nonspecific lumbar epidural steroid injections. This is performed by inserting an epidural needle through the sacral hiatus into epidural space at the sacral canal.

Most pain specialists prefer to use fluoroscopic guidance for positioning of the epidural needle, as a blind injection may result in 30% to 40% needle misplacement. Fluoroscopic guidance with radiographic contrast also allows for documentation of the appropriate placement of epidural steroids to improve safety, accuracy, and potential efficacy.

Clinical studies of epidural steroid injections

There have been more than 70 studies on epidural steroids reported in world literature. Although many studies prove the short-term benefits of epidural steroid injections, the long-term benefits are less convincing. Because of the differing results with various techniques performed by a wide range of specialists, the effectiveness of epidural steroid injections continues to be a topic of debate. Koes, Watts, and McQuay performed systematic reviews and meta-analyses on many of the pertinent studies and found conflicting results [37–40]. In 2003, Aldrete performed a prospective study comparing Indomethacin injection (not currently used clinically) with Methylprednisolone in 206 patients. The study found a reduction in pain on the Visual Analog Scale, increased physical activity, reduction in emotional distress, and a reduced intake of medication in all groups. The study also determined that 2 mg of Indomethacin were better than 1 mg, and equivalent to 80 mg of Methylprednisolone [41].

Studies have demonstrated positive efficacy of lumbar ESIs when proper placement is confirmed by using fluoroscopic guidance and radiographic confirmation through the use of contrast. Approximately 60% to 75% of patients receive some relief after ESIs. Benefits include relief of radicular and low back pain, with leg pain more improved than low back pain; increased quality of life; reduced need for pain medicine; improved work status; and decreased requirements for hospitalization and surgery. Studies have determined that patients who have symptoms for fewer than 3 months have response rates of 90%. Those who have symptoms for fewer than 6 months have response rates of 70%, and those who have symptoms over a year have response rates of only 50% [42,43]. Abdi and colleagues recently concluded that there is moderate evidence for interlaminar epidurals in the cervical spine and limited evidence in the lumbar spine for long-term relief [44]. The evidence for cervical and lumbar transforaminal epidural steroid injections is moderate for long-term improvement in managing nerve root pain [44]. The evidence for caudal epidural steroid injections is moderate for long-term relief in managing nerve root pain and chronic low back pain.

Selective nerve root blocks

Selective nerve root blocks may be used both for diagnostic purposes [45] and pain relief. These blocks provide useful information for patients who have radiculopathy but have not had successful or concordant diagnoses by means of imaging studies or electromyogram (EMG). A positive result includes immediate worsening or improvement of symptoms or long-term improvement of pain with corticosteroids. Selective nerve root blocks also may be performed for therapeutic purposes to treat degenerative changes of the spine with referred pain and intraneural edema inflammation related to herniated discs. Selective transforaminal nerve root steroid injections have several advantages over nonselective ESIs. Theses include diagnostic capability, closer proximity to the specific pain source, smaller volumes of injectate, and lower risks of intrathecal steroid injection.

Posterior procedure for selective lumbar transforaminal nerve root injection

Selective nerve blocks most commonly are performed with fluoroscopic guidance and the patient in the prone position, although they also may be approached obliquely. The fluoroscope should be positioned to line up the spinous processes with the center of the vertebral body with the superior endplate pictured in tangent. The position inferior to the transverse process and lateral to the facet joint should be determined and marked and then the spin prepared and draped sterilely. A curve of approximately 30° should be made at the distal end of a 22-gauge spinal needle, with the bevel on the outside of the curve. After local infiltration, the needle should be advanced, keeping the tip lateral to the facet joint, continually confirming depth of the needle by means of fluoroscopic rotation and confirmation. When the projection, the needle tip should be directed medially using the 30° curve and appropriate torque toward the midline of the pedicle on an anteroposterior projection and the anterior foramen on the lateral projection (Fig. 4). If paresthesias are encountered, the needle advancement should be ceased to avoid nerve injury. When the needle has reached this position, a small amount of contrast should be injected to confirm needle placement followed by the desired injectate [46–48].

For diagnostic purposes, the injectate may be 1% lidocaine with or without bupivacaine. Examples of an injectate used for therapeutic purposes include 0.5 to 1 mL or less of a steroid, betamethasone (Celestone) 6 mg or methylprednisolone (Depo-Medrol) 80 mg, mixed with 0.5 mL of bupivacaine. A small total volume should be used to prevent the spread of anesthetic to adjacent nerve roots or into the epidural space, particularly if the block is performed for its diagnostic utility.

Clinical studies of selective nerve root blocks with steroids

Riew and colleagues [49] performed a prospective, randomized, controlled, double-blinded study of patients who initially were deemed surgical candidates and initially desired surgery to improve symptoms of radiculopathy. After undergoing a selective nerve block with steroid and local anesthetic, approximately 71% of patients elected not to undergo surgery. Most studies report pain relief for approximately 1 to 3 months in patients who have initial pain improvement, although some studies have found even longer durations for pain relief [45,47–49].

Open surgical treatment for painful sciatica

When conservative measures and minimally invasive measures fail, patients often resort to surgery. Surgical decompression first was popularized

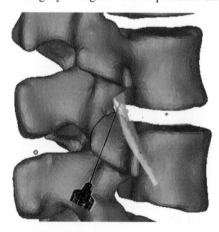

Fig. 4. Selective nerve root block. The needle is positioned into the neuroforamen with fluoroscopic guidance.

by Dandy, Mixter, and Barr [50,51]. A lumbar discectomy once mandated a complete lumbar laminectomy. Currently, a microdiscectomy by any method has become the operation of choice. Despite the fact that patients who undergo decompression will have a more rapid resolution of symptoms, long-term results are no different than when compared with nonoperative management as proven by Weber [52]. More recently, Peul and colleagues randomly assigned 283 patients who had a diagnosis of severe incapacitating lumbosacral syndrome from an attending neurologist lasting for 6 to 12 weeks to early surgery versus prolonged conservative treatment (with eventual surgery if needed) [53]. They concluded that the 1-year outcomes were similar for patients assigned to early surgery and those assigned to conservative treatment, but the rates of pain relief and of perceived recovery were faster for those assigned to early surgery [53]. With this being the case, attempts at injections rather than surgery would seem a logical choice.

Minimally invasive techniques for the treatment of lumbar spinal stenosis

Spinal stenosis may congenital, acquired through the degenerative process, or a combination of both. The degenerative changes that may contribute to spinal stenosis include disc failure with herniation, spinal ligament buckling and hypertrophy, facet joint degeneration, and spondylolisthesis. All of these degenerative changes may result in central spinal canal narrowing. Although patients who have lumbosacral radicular pain suffer with isolated compression along with inflammation at an individual nerve root, lumbar spinal stenosis describes constriction of all of the nerve roots that pass a larger area of constriction that has developed over time. Spinal stenosis is most common at L3-4, L4-5, and L5-S1 [8].

Despite tremendous technological advances in medical imaging, the diagnosis of lumbar spinal stenosis remains clinical. It is diagnosed primarily by a thorough history and later confirmed by imaging such as an MRI or CT myelogram. Patients who have lumbar stenosis often present with radiating leg pain associated with walking that is relieved by rest. This is referred to as neurogenic claudication. Patients may report that bending forward diminishes the pain. Patients often report improved symptoms leaning over a shopping cart. A characteristic symptom is an improvement of pain walking up stairs and a worsening of symptoms walking down them. This finding is attributed to the dynamic element that may be present in lumbar spinal stenosis. In the flexed position, there is a relative increase in the size of the spinal canal. This fact recently has become the basis of an innovative minimally invasive method used to treat lumbar spinal stenosis [54].

Conservative treatment

Treatment with conservative measures may provide relief for patients who have mild symptoms; however, as with cervical spinal stenosis, the role of conservative treatment for those who are severely stenotic is limited. Treatment may consist of nonsteroidal anti-inflammatory drugs (NSAIDs), physical therapy, and education. These initial measures may be useful for patients who have mild symptoms. All of these treatments are directed at ameliorating the patient symptoms and are often regrettably of finite use, because they do not address the patient's underlying spinal stenosis. As with any medical intervention, treatment should be tailored to the patient. Patients who have significant morbidity and extremely short life expectancy are poor candidates for a large decompression [27].

Epidural steroid injections

ESIs are offered to treat the component of the patient's leg pain attributed to nerve inflammation. The technique and clinical results of epidural steroids are reviewed previously. The results of studies vary in the literature as to the true usefulness of epidural steroids for spinal syndromes such as lumbar stenosis, with most studies finding injection techniques more useful at controlling discrete leg pain. Although high-level evidence is sparse that epidural injections will improve clinical symptoms such as walking intolerance from neurogenic claudication, it may remain an option for those patients for whom conservative treatment is most appropriate [55].

Surgical treatment

Traditionally, when surgical interventions are considered, the entirety of the offending areas of compression should be removed. This entails a posterior spine decompression with an extensive laminectomy and partial facetectomy. Instability may result from the decompression, necessitating spinal fusion along with instrumentation. Spinal instability may contribute to the patient's stenosis, as is the case in patients who have symptomatic spondylolisthesis. In addition to any degenerative changes or congenital stenosis, the translation of the vertebral bodies seen in patients who have spondylolisthesis further narrows the spinal canal. Patients also may possess dynamic spondylolisthesis where the vertebral translation is not fixed and occurs with flexion/extension of the lumbar spine. Either of these cases contributes to the need for a fusion procedure in addition to a decompression. Novel alternative systems to traditional rigid fusions such as Anatomic Facet Replacement System (AFRS), which allows more physiologic spinal movements, are being investigated for the lumbar region.

X stop

An innovative alternative to decompressive lumbar surgery has come into use and has achieved a great deal of attention in the lay press. The X Stop (Kyphon, Sunnyvale, California) device was approved by the FDA in November of 2005. As discussed earlier in the article, the cross-sectional area at one segment of the spine can increase as much as 50% from extension to flexion [55]. This relative size increase is felt to explain why patients note improvement in their symptoms when ascending stairs or leaning over a shopping cart. X Stop attempts to recreate this flexion surgically.

For the procedure, patients often are placed in the lateral position. This positioning serves two purposes. First, by being lateral rather than prone, patients place their spine in a position of relative flexion, which is necessary for device placement. The lateral position also allows for the drainage of blood from the surgical field. Surgeons also may choose to perform the procedure with the patient in the prone position, using bolsters or table modifications to create a relative flexed position of the spine. The lateral position is preferred by most and is recommended by the manufacturer [56].

A small posterior skin incision is made at the level of symptomatic stenosis, which is localized at the time of surgery with a fluoroscope or other form of radiographic guidance. The dissection continues until the spinous processes of the symptomatic levels are exposed. The spacer component of the device then is placed between the spinous processes. There are two buttresses on either side of the oval spacer that prevent migration. The isolated motion segment then is held in a relatively flexed position by the spacer, while the adjacent levels are allowed to freely flex and extend. The titanium metal implant fits between the spinous processes of the vertebrae without any attachment to the patient's bones or ligaments (Fig. 5). As patient anatomy varies, the oval spacer comes in sizes varying from 6 to 16 mm. Size selection depends on the size of implant required to maintain adequate flexion at the symptomatic motion segment.

The primary advantage of the device is its minimally invasive approach for implantation. The device is useful if the stenotic area of the spine encompassed one or two spinal levels. Early clinical trials have found good efficacy and excellent safety profiles. In a multicenter study, 100 patients with lumbar spinal stenosis who underwent the X Stop procedure were compared with 91 patients who were treated conservatively. At 2 years of follow-up, approximately half of the patients who underwent the X Stop experienced statistically significant improvement in pain relief and activity level. Patients who have undergone an X Stop procedure remain candidates for surgical decompression for persistent or recurrent symptoms [57].

Minimally invasive techniques for the treatment of compression fractures

More than half of Americans over the age of 50 suffer from either osteopenia or osteoporosis, with approximately 700,000 vertebral compression fractures occurring annually. Women are affected disproportionately making up over 75% of the fracture population [58,59]. Vertebral compression fractures exact an often unmeasured toll with patients who sustain vertebral compression fractures suffering from both acute and chronic pain and

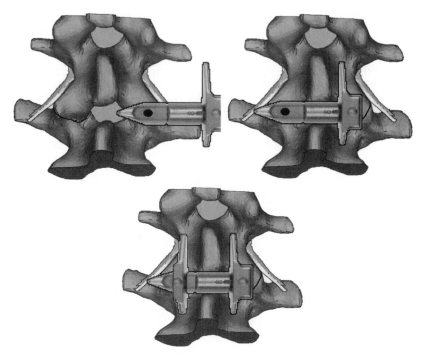

Fig. 5. The X-Stop (Kyphon, Sunnyvale, California) device consists of a spacer that is placed surgically between the spinous processes. Once the spacer is placed, a second buttress is attached to the implant, preventing migration.

progressive kyphosis [60,61]. The effects of multiple vertebral fractures may bear the added morbidity of weight loss because of early satiety, poor psychological well-being, and pulmonary complications such as decreased pulmonary function. Although these fractures are rarely a direct cause of death, they frequently produce very significant morbidities that eventually may affect mortality [12–19,62–72]. Attempts at surgical interventions have been fraught with disaster both because of implant failure from poor bone stock, and mortality because of the poor general health of the patients undergoing surgery.

Percutaneous vertebral augmentation

In the 1960s, Sir John Charnley introduced the orthopedic community to the use of polymethylmethacrylate (PMMA) for total hip replacement [73,74]. In the spine, PMMA first was used to treat a painful and aggressive variant of a vertebral hemangioma [75–78]. The technique later was used to treat painful metastases to the vertebral body [79]. Thermal necrosis has been proposed as the primary method of action for the pain relief provided by both vertebroplasty and kyphoplasty [80]. The polymerization reaction of PMMA cement is exothermic and can reach up to 122°C [80,81].

Conservative therapy consisting of oral nonsteroidal medications and opioid analgesia should be offered initially. Patients are offered a spinal orthosis in addition to their pain medication. Injured osteoporotic patients are at risk of significant medical morbidity the longer they remain immobile. Early percutaneous vertebral augmentation may be offered to patients who have a documented inability to mobilize after their injury; however, patents typically are given 4 to 6 weeks to improve [60].

Vertebral fractures with cortical disruption that would preclude cement containment as determined on preoperative CT or MRI images should not undergo a percutaneous vertebral augmentation. Vertebra that are collapsed completely are difficult if not impossible to augment [82]. Fracture acuity has been found to be a determinant of treatment results. Bone scan and STIR-weighted MRI are useful in determining fracture acuity, as patients often have had previous fractures in the distant past that may be obvious on a radiographic image but inconsequential in the patient's current clinical state of back pain.

There are numerous anesthesia choices for percutaneous vertebral augmentation. Local anesthesia may be selected. The local anesthetic is injected into the skin, subcutaneous tissues, and periosteum of the vertebra. Conscious sedation often is offered as an adjuvant. General anesthesia is another possible choice.

Vertebroplasty

The first vertebroplasty was performed for an aggressive C2 hemangioma in Amiens, France, in 1984 [83]. Use of this technique later was introduced to the United States by interventional neuroradiologists at the University of Virginia, and it has gained increasing popularity with patients reporting rapid pain relief [84].

The procedure level is verified on the preoperative imaging and finally on the image intensifier before needle/cannula placement. After localization, a small incision is made, and an 11-gauge cannulated trocar and bone biopsy needle is passed under fluoroscopic guidance. The cannula is passed through the pedicle into the vertebral body being treated. Both lateral and anteroposterior projections provide necessary visualization of the path of the needle. An alternative approach is parapedicular. This approach most often is used to access the thoracic spine. The parapedicular approach involves inserting the cannula between the lateral margin of the pedicle of thoracic vertebrae and the rib head [75].

Before injection of the cement, a vertebrogram may be performed to identify the basivertebral venous plexus and other large vessels that are susceptible for extravasation [85]. Additionally, it is suggested that 30% wt/vol of pure barium sulfate be added to the PMMA powder before mixing so as to allow imaging of the cement during injection. Alternate imaging techniques may be used. Biplane fluoroscopy will allow visualization in two planes during injection and often is chosen when the procedure is performed in a radiology department because of equipment availability and familiarity. CT guidance also may be used. Similar to the image-guided techniques described earlier, however, CT adds more to the cost and radiation exposure of the procedure than is often necessary. Cement injection must be complete within 6 to 8 minutes before it becomes too viscous [73].

The patient should be observed for 1 to 3 hours after operation. Pain relief is usually immediate. Follow-up radiographs may be indicated if the patient fails to respond positively to the intervention, as an incorrect level may have been treated, or a new fracture may have occurred after the vertebroplasty procedure [86].

Numerous studies have demonstrated the effectiveness of vertebroplasty. Grados and colleagues [87] found significant pain improvement based on a visual analog scale within 1 month that was still improved at a mean follow-up of 2 years. Zoarski and colleagues [88] found significant improvement in pain, disability, physical function, and psychological well being. On the other hand, other studies have found up to a 10% failure rate for the procedure [89].

Unique complications to vertebroplasty and kyphoplasty include cement extravasation and fracture of vertebral bodies adjacent to the levels treated. The rate of cement extravasation has been reported as up to 6% for vertebral level treated; however, the rate of neural symptoms from such leakage has been reported between 0% and 4% [60]. Specific technical safeguards and the use of contrast within the cement mixture are ways to prevent the most frequent complication of percutaneous vertebral augmentation.

Kyphoplasty

The possibility of cement extravasation, although low, poses devastating neurologic consequences. The high pressures used to introduce the cement also potentially could cause bolus embolization of cement through the venous channels to the lungs. The kyphoplasty technique provided a possible answer to these concerns and provided a means to attempt a fracture reduction. Kyphoplasty first was performed in 1998 [90]. The procedure has achieved the same pain relief as vertebroplasty.

The kyphoplasty technique is performed in a similar manner as vertebroplasty. Fluoroscopic guidance is used to identify the fracture site. A 1 cm incision is made just lateral to both pedicles of the vertebral body to be treated. A Jamshidi needle (Kyphon, Sunnyvale, California) is used to enter the superior lateral border of the pedicle. Under fluoroscopic guidance, the Jamshidi needle is passed through the pedicle into the vertebral body. Once the Jamshidi needle enters the vertebral body, the needle is exchanged for an obturator (Kyphon) . This is followed by placement of a working cannula (Kyphon). A drill then is used to create a tract into the vertebral body. The balloon catheter finally is placed into the fracture, and the entire process is repeated on the contralateral side. Both balloon tamps (Kyphon) are inflated simultaneously. Once the fracture is reduced, the balloons are removed. The voids created by the balloons are filled under low pressure with methyl methacrylate cement using a hand plunger system supplied by the manufacturer (Fig. 6). Intraoperative radiographs are used to confirm containment of the cement in the vertebral body [86].

The pain relief provided by kyphoplasty appears similar to that reported for vertebroplasty. The first long-term data reported on kyphoplasty in 2001 found that 95% of patients treated with kyphoplasty or vertebroplasty had significant improvement in pain [60,90]. Also, Lieberman and colleagues published the results of a phase 1 study of the inflatable bone tamp technique used in the kyphoplasty procedure that showed significant improvement in pain scores and physical function ($P = .0001$) [64]. In a multicenter study, almost all patients treated by kyphoplasty were able to return to their baseline activities and wean themselves off of opioid medications [90].

Fracture reduction also has been a proposed advantage of kyphoplasty over vertebroplasty. The reported percent vertebral height restoration has ranged between 30% and 86%, with a reduction in relative kyphosis reported between 5% and 13% [62,91–94].

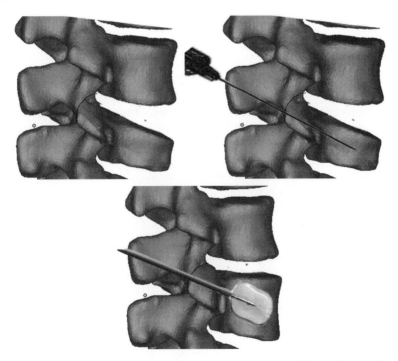

Fig. 6. Percutaneous vertebral augmentation. Both vertebroplasty and kyphoplasty involve the injection of bone cement through the pedicle of a vertebra that has sustained a compression fracture. Kyphoplasty involves the addition of a balloon tamp to possibly reduce the fracture and create a void for cement injection.

Crandall and colleagues [93] found the greatest degree of height correction and a disparity between the treatment results of old and new fractures. The height restoration of 86% was reported for what were termed as new or acute fractures, while the authors reported that fractures that were subacute (older than 4 months) had a 79% correction. The kyphotic angle correction differed based on fracture age also. Kyphoplasty of new fractures resulted in a 7° correction, while subacute fractures were reduced by 5°.

For patients who underwent one- to three-level kyphoplasty procedures, measurements revealed that kyphoplasty reduced local kyphotic deformity at the fractured vertebra by an average of 7.3°. Overall angular correction decreased to 2.4° (20% of preoperative kyphosis at fractured level) when measured one level above and below. The angular correction further decreased to 1.5° and 1.0° (13% and 8% of preoperative kyphosis at fractured level), respectively, at spans of two and three levels above and below. With multilevel kyphoplasty procedures, the total gains seen over multiple vertebrae such as 7.8° over two levels and 7.7° over three levels compared with the 7.3° for a single level. In other words, the small correction in fracture height and angulation achieved through the use of kyphoplasty does not translate into a substantial improvement in the general sagittal alignment of the spine as a whole [62].

Summary

Numerous interventional techniques offer patients an alternative to either continued and possibly futile conservative management or perhaps a large surgical procedure. Facet blocks, epidural steroid injections, selective nerve root injections, and discography/IDET may provide a possible means of treating back pain with or without lower extremity symptoms. Definitive data supporting or refuting the long-term effectiveness of these procedures over years are uncertain, however. In addition, X Stop has now offered an alternative for patients with mild lumbar stenosis. Kyphoplasty and vertebroplasty have offered patients who have painful compression fractures a means of treatment that could allow them to return to their activities with a measurable improvement in their pain. Kyphoplasty may offer the possibility of fracture reduction. There is no magic bullet in the treatment of spine-related pain, but these techniques may offer some hope for older persons who have intractable back pain. Furthermore, these techniques may be particularly well-suited for a subpopulation of older persons who do not tolerate pharmacologic treatment options well.

References

[1] van Tulder M, Koes B. Low back pain (chronic). Clin Evid 2006;15:1634–53.

[2] Andersson GBJ. The epidemiology of spinal disorders. In: Frymoyer JW, editor. The adult spine: principles and practice. 2nd edition. New York: Raven Press; 1997. p. 93–141.

[3] Frymoyer JW. Back pain and sciatica. N Engl J Med 1988;318(5):291–300.

[4] Macfarlane GJ. Who will develop chronic pain and why? In: Flor H, Kalso E, Dostrovsky JO, editors. The epidemiological evidence proceedings of the 11th World Congress on Pain. Seattle (WA): International Association for the Study of Pain (IASP) Press; 2006.

[5] Koes BW, van Tulder MW, Thomas S. Diagnosis and treatment of low back pain. BMJ 2006;332(7555):1430–4.

[6] Deyo RA, Rainville J, Kent DL. What can the history and physical examination tell us about low back pain? J Am Med Assoc 1992;268(6):760–5.

[7] Adams MA, Roughley PJ. What is intervertebral disc degeneration, and what causes it? Spine 2006;31(18):2151–61.

[8] Garfin SR, Rydevik BL, Lipson SJ. Spinal stenosis: pathophysiology. In: Herkowitz H, Garfin SR, Balderson RA, et al, editors. The spine. 4th edition. Philadelphia: W.B. Saunders Co.; 1999. p. 791–826.

[9] Kirkaldy-Willis WH, Wedge JH, Yong-Hing K, et al. Pathology and pathogenesis of lumbar spondylosis and stenosis. Spine 1978;3(4):319–28.

[10] Crock HV. A reappraisal of intervertebral disc lesions. Med J Aust 1970;1(20):983–9.

[11] Merskey H, Bogduk N. Classification of chronic pain: descriptions of chronic pain syndromes and definitions of pain terms. Seattle (WA): IASP Press; 1994. p. 180–1.

[12] Ahmed M, Bjurholm A, Kreicbergs A, et al. Neuropeptide Y, tyrosine hydroxylase, and vasoactive intestinal polypeptide-immunoreactive nerve fibers in the vertebral bodies, discs, dura mater, and spinal ligaments of the rat lumbar spine. Spine 1993;18:268–73.

[13] Hirsch C. An attempt to diagnose the level of a disc lesion clinically by disc puncture. Acta Orthop 1948;18:132–40.

[14] Tomecek FJ, Anthony CS, Boxell C, et al. Discography interpretation and techniques in the lumbar spine. Neurosurg Focus 2002;13(2):1–8.

[15] Lindblom K. Diagnostic puncture of intervertebral discs in sciatia. Acta Orthop Scand 1948; 17:231–9.

[16] Guyer RD, Ohnmeiss DD. Contemporary concepts in spine care—lumbar discography. Spine 1995;20(18):2048–59.

[17] Fraser RD, Osti OL, Vernon-Roberts B. Discitis after discography. J Bone Joint Surg Br 1987;69B(1):26–35.

[18] Guyer RD, Collier R, Stith WJ, et al. Discitis after discography. Spine 1988;13(12):1352–4.

[19] Gill K, Blumenthal SL. Functional results after anterior lumbar fusion at L5–S1 in patients with normal and abnormal MRI scans. Spine 1992;17:940–2.

[20] Buenaventura RM, Shah RV, Patel V, et al. Systematic review of discography as a diagnostic test for spinal pain: an update. Pain Physician 2007;10(1):147–64.

[21] Lechter F, Goldring S. The effect of radiofrequency current and heat on peripheral nerve action potential in the cat. J Neurosurg 1968;29:42–7.

[22] Smith H, McWhorter J, Challa V. Radiofrequency neurolysis in a clinical model: neuropathological correlation. J Neurosurg 1981;55:246–53.

[23] Available at: http://idet.msltechdev.com/2000_professional/. Accessed October 2007.

[24] Andersson GB, Mekhail NA, Block JE. Treatment of intractable discogenic low back pain. A systematic review of spinal fusion and intradiscal electrothermal therapy (IDET). Pain Physician 2006;9(3):237–48.

[25] Urrutia G, Kovacs F, Nishishinya MB, et al. Percutaneous thermocoagulation intradiscal techniques for discogenic low back pain. Spine 2007;32(10):1146–54.

[26] Boswell MV, Colson JD, Sehgal N, et al. A systematic review of therapeutic facet joint interventions in chronic spinal pain. Pain Physician 2007;10(1):229–53.

[27] Lavelle W, Carl A, Lavelle ED. Invasive and minimally invasive surgical techniques for back pain conditions. Med Clin North Am 2007;91(2):287–98.

[28] Cornefjord M, Olmarker K, Farley DB, et al. Neuropeptide changes in compressed spinal nerve roots. Spine 1995;20(6):670–3.

[29] Rydevik B, Brown MD, Lundborg G. Pathoanatomy and pathophysiology of nerve root compression. Spine 1984;9(1):7–15.

[30] Takebayashi T, Cavanaugh JM, Cuneyt Ozaktay A, et al. Effect of nucleus pulposus on the neural activity of dorsal root ganglion. Spine 2001;26(8):940–5.

[31] Adams MA, Bogduk N, Burton K, et al. The biomechanics of back pain. Edinburgh (UK): Churchill Livingstone; 2002.

[32] Trout JJ, Buckwalter JA, Moore KC. Ultrastructure of the human intervertebral disc. II. Cells of the nucleus pulposus. Anat Rec 1982;204(4):307–14.

[33] Boswell MV, Trescot AM, Datta S, et al. Interventional techniques: evidence-based practice guidelines in the management of chronic spinal pain. Pain Physician 2007;10(1):7–111.

[34] Burkle CM, Sands RP, Bacon DR, et al. Beyond blocks: the history of the development of techniques in regional anesthesia. In Raj PP. editor. Textbook of regional anesthesia New York: Churchill Livingstone; 2002. p. 27.

[35] Olsson SE. The dynamic factor in spinal cord compression. J Neurosurg 1958;15:308–21.

[36] Davidson JT, Robin GC. Epidural injections in the lumbosciatic syndrome. Br J Anaesth 1961;33:595–8.

[37] Koes BW, Scholten RPM, Mens JMA, et al. Efficacy of epidural steroid injections for low back pain and sciatica: a systematic review of randomized clinical trials. Pain 1995;63: 279–88.

[38] Koes BW, Scholten JPM, Mens JMA, et al. Epidural steroid injections for low back pain and sciatica: an updated systematic review of randomized clinical trials. Pain Digest 1999;9: 241–7.

[39] Watts RW, Silagy CA. A meta-analysis on the efficacy of epidural corticosteroids in the treatment of sciatica. Anaesth Intensive Care 1995;23:564–9.

[40] McQuay HJ, Moore RA. An evidence-based resource for pain relief. London: Oxford University Press; 1998.

[41] Aldrete JA. Epidural injections of indomethacin for postlaminectomy syndrome: a preliminary report. Anesth Analg 2003;96(2):463–8.

[42] Botwin KP, Gruber RD, Bouchlas CG, et al. Fluoroscopically guided lumbar transforaminal epidural steroid injections in degenerative lumbar stenosis: an outcome study. Am J Phys Med Rehabil 2002;81(12):898–905.

[43] el-Khoury GY, Ehara S, Weinstein JN, et al. Epidural steroid injection: a procedure ideally performed with fluoroscopic control. Radiology 1988;168(2):554–7.

[44] Abdi S, Datta S, Trescot AM, et al. Epidural steroids in the management of chronic spinal pain: a systematic review. Pain Physician 2007;10(1):185–212.

[45] Datta S, Everett CR, Trescot AM, et al. An updated systematic review of the diagnostic utility of selective nerve root blocks. Pain Physician 2007;10(1):113–28.

[46] Dooley JF, McBroom RJ, Taguchi T, et al. Nerve root infiltration in the diagnosis of radicular pain. Spine 1988;13(1):79–83.

[47] Link SC, el-Khoury GY, Guilford WB. Percutaneous epidural and nerve root block and percutaneous lumbar sympatholysis. Radiol Clin North Am 1998;36(3):509–21.

[48] Murtagh R. The art and science of nerve root and facet blocks. Neuroimaging Clin N Am 2000;10(3):465–77.

[49] Riew KD, Park JB, Cho YS, et al. Nerve root blocks in the treatment of lumbar radicular pain. A minimum five-year follow-up. J Bone Joint Surg Am 2006;88(8):1722–5.

[50] Dandy WE. Loose cartilage from intervertebral disk simulating tumor of the spinal cord. By Walter E. Dandy, 1929. Clin Orthop Relat Res 1989;238:4–8.

[51] Wisneski RJ, Garfin SR, Rothman RH. Lumbar disc disease. In: Herkowitz H, Garfin SR, Balderson RA, et al, editors. The spine. 4th edition. Philadelphia: W.B. Saunders Co.; 1999. p. 671–746.

[52] Weber H. The natural history of disc herniation and the influence of intervention. Spine 1994;19(19):2234–8.

[53] Peul WC, van Houwlingen HC, van den Hour WB, et al. Surgery versus prolonged conservative treatment for sciatica. N Engl J Med 2007;356(22):2245–56.

[54] Richards J, Majumdar S, Lindsey DP, et al. The treatment mechanism of an interspinous process implant for lumbar neurogenic intermittent claudication. Spine 2005; 30(7):744–9.

[55] Boswell MV, Hansen HC, Trescot AM, et al. Epidural steroids in the management of chronic spinal pain and radiculopathy. Pain Physician 2003;6(3):319–34.

[56] Kyphon: What is the X-STOP® IPD® System? Available at: http://www.kyphon.com/sfmt/press/xstop.html. Accessed October 2007.

[57] Zucherman JF, Hsu KY, Hartjen CA, et al. A multicenter, prospective, randomized trial evaluating the X Stop interspinous process decompression system for the treatment of neurogenic intermittent claudication: two-year follow-up results. Spine 2005;30(12):1351–8.

[58] Lemke DM. Vertebroplasty and kyphoplasty for treatment of painful osteoporotic compression fractures. J Am Acad Nurse Pract 2005;17(7):268–76.

[59] National Osteoporosis Foundation. 2005 annual report. Available at: http://www.nof.org/aboutnof/2005_Annual_Report_FINAL.pdf. Accessed December 20, 2006.

[60] Truumees E, Hilibrand A, Vaccaro AR. Percutaneous vertebral augmentation. Spine J 2004; 4(2):218–29.

[61] Wasnich U. Vertebral fracture epidemiology. Bone 1996;18:1791–6.

[62] Pradhan BB, Bae HW, Kropf MA, et al. Kyphoplasty reduction of osteoporotic vertebral compression fractures: correction of local kyphosis versus overall sagittal alignment. Spine 2006;31(4):435–41.

[63] Schlaich C, Minne HW, Bruckner T, et al. Reduced pulmonary function in patients with spinal osteoporotic fractures. Osteoporos Int 1998;8(3):261–7.

[64] Leech JA, Dulberg C, Kellie S, et al. Relationship of lung function to severity of osteoporosis in women. Am Rev Respir Dis 1990;141(1):68–71.

[65] Leidig-Bruckner G, Minne HW, Schlaich C, et al. Clinical grading of spinal osteoporosis: quality of life components and spinal deformity in women with chronic low back pain and women with vertebral osteoporosis. J Bone Miner Res 1997;12(4):663–75.

[66] Kado DM, Duong T, Stone KL, et al. Incident vertebral fractures and mortality in older women: a prospective study. Osteoporos Int 2003;14(7):589–94.

[67] Jalava T, Sarna S, Pylkkanen L, et al. Association between vertebral fracture and increased mortality in osteoporotic patients. J Bone Miner Res 2003;18(7):1254–60.

[68] Silverman SL, Delmas PD, Kulkarni PM, et al. Comparison of fracture, cardiovascular event, and breast cancer rates at 3 years in postmenopausal women with osteoporosis. J Am Geriatr Soc 2004;52(9):1543–8.

[69] Cooper C, Atkinson EJ, Jacobsen SJ, et al. Population-based study of survival after osteoporotic fractures. Am J Epidemiol 1993;137:1001–5.

[70] Ismail AA, O'Neill TW, Cooper C, et al. Mortality associated with vertebral deformity in men and women: results from the European Prospective Osteoporosis Study (EPOS). Osteoporos Int 1998;8:291–7.

[71] Ensrud K, Thompson D, Cauley J, et al. Prevalent vertebral deformities predict mortality and hospitalization in older women with low bone mass. J Am Geriatr Soc 2000;48:241–9.

[72] Cauley JA, Thompson DE, Ensrud KC, et al. Risk of mortality following clinical fractures. Osteoporos Int 2000;11:556–61.

[73] Mathis JM, Maroney M, Fenton DC, et al. Evaluation of bone cements for use in percutaneous vertebroplasty [abstract]. Proceedings of the 13th Annual Meeting of the North American Spine Society 1998:210–1.

[74] DiMaio FR. The science of bone cement: a historical review. Orthopedics 2002;25(12): 1399–407.

[75] Hide IG, Gangi A. Percutaneous vertebroplasty: history, technique and current perspectives. Clin Radiol 2004;59:461–7.

[76] Cortet B, Cotten A, Deprez X, et al. Value of vertebroplasty combined with surgical decompression in the treatment of aggressive spinal angioma. Apropos of 3 cases. Rev Rhum Ed Fr 1994;61(1):16–22.

[77] Ide C, Gangi A, Rimmelin A, et al. Vertebral haemangiomas with spinal cord compression: the place of preoperative percutaneous vertebroplasty with methyl methacrylate. Neuroradiology 1996;38(6):585–9.

[78] Feydy A, Cognard C, Miaux Y, et al. Acrylic vertebroplasty in symptomatic cervical vertebral haemangiomas: report of 2 cases. Neuroradiology 1996;38(4):389–91.

[79] Weill A, Chiras J, Simon JM, et al. Spinal metastases: indications for and results of percutaneous injection of acrylic surgical cement. Radiology 1996;199(1):241–7.

[80] Jefferiss CD, Lee AJC, Ling RSM. Thermal aspects of self-curing polymethylmethacrylate. J Bone Joint Surg Br 1975;57B(4):511–8.

[81] Danilewicz-Stysiak Z. Experimental investigations on the cytotoxic nature of methyl methacrylate. J Prosthet Dent 1980;44(1):13–6.

[82] Barr JD, Barr MS, Lemley TJ, et al. Percutaneous vertebroplasty for pain relief and spinal stabilization. Spine 2000;25(8):923–8.

[83] Galibert P, Deramond H, Rosat P, et al. Preliminary note on the treatment of vertebral angioma by percutaneous acrylic vertebroplasty. Neurochirurgie 1987;33:166–8.

[84] Jensen ME, Evans AJ, Mathis JM, et al. Percutaneous polymethylmethacrylate vertebroplasty in the treatment of osteoporotic vertebral body compression fractures: technical aspects. AJNR Am J Neuroradiol 1997;18(10):1897–904.

[85] Gaughen JR Jr, Jensen ME, Schweickert PA, et al. Relevance of antecedent venography in percutaneous vertebroplasty for the treatment of osteoporotic compression fractures. AJNR Am J Neuroradiol 2002;23(4):594–600.

[86] Lavelle WF, Cheney R. Recurrent fracture after vertebral kyphoplasty. Spine J 2006;6(5): 488–93.

[87] Grados F, Depriester C, Cayrolle G, et al. Long-term observations of vertebral osteoporotic fractures treated by percutaneous vertebroplasty. Rheumatology (Oxford) 2000;39:1410–4.

[88] Zoarski GH, Snow P, Olan WJ, et al. Percutaneous vertebroplasty for osteoporotic compression fractures: quantitative prospective evaluation of long-term outcomes. J Vasc Interv Radiol 2002;13:139–48.

[89] Armsen N, Boszczyk B. Vertebro-/kyphoplasty history, development, results. European Journal of Trauma and Emergency Surgery 2005;5:433–41.

[90] Garfin SR, Yuan HA, Reiley MA. New technologies in spine: kyphoplasty and vertebroplasty for the treatment of painful osteoporotic compression fractures. Spine 2001;26(14): 1511–5.

[91] Boszczyk BM, Bierschneider M, Schmid K, et al. Microsurgical interlaminary vertebro- and kyphoplasty for severe osteoporotic fractures. J Neurosurg 2004;100(Suppl 1):32–7.

[92] Lieberman IH, Dudeney S, Reinhardt MK, et al. Initial outcome and efficacy of kyphoplasty in the treatment of painful osteoporotic vertebral compression fractures. Spine 2001;26(14): 1631–8.

[93] Crandall D, Slaughter D, Hankins PJ, et al. Acute versus chronic vertebral compression fractures treated with kyphoplasty: early results. Spine J 2004;4(4):418–24.

[94] Ledlie JT, Renfro M. Balloon kyphoplasty: one-year outcomes in vertebral body height restoration, chronic pain, and activity levels. J Neurosurg 2003;98(Suppl 1):36–42.

ELSEVIER
SAUNDERS

CLINICS IN
GERIATRIC
MEDICINE

Clin Geriatr Med 24 (2008) 369–388

Lumbar Spinal Stenosis in Older Adults: Current Understanding and Future Directions

John D. Markman, MD[a],*, Kristina G. Gaud, BS[b]

[a]*Neuromedicine Pain Management Center, University of Rochester School of Medicine and Dentistry, Department of Neurosurgery, 601 Elmwood Avenue, Box 670, Rochester, NY 14642, USA*
[b]*University of Rochester School of Medicine and Dentistry, Department of Neurosurgery, 601 Elmwood Avenue, Rochester, NY 14642, USA*

Lumbar spinal stenosis is a common cause of low back pain and the leading indication for lumbar surgery in the United States for persons over 65 years of age [1]. Neurogenic intermittent claudication is the hallmark of the clinical syndrome of lumbar spinal stenosis. This distinctive pattern of pain in the back and legs is induced by erect postures, such as when standing or walking. Neurogenic intermittent claudication is a major cause of impaired mobility and loss of independence in seniors [2].

The advent of axial imaging technologies has increased the sensitivity of diagnostic testing for lumbar spinal stenosis over the past three decades [3]. These tools offer precise anatomic characterization of spinal structures, but understanding of the pathophysiology of neurogenic claudication has lagged far behind. Pain medications are prescribed widely for treatment of neurogenic intermittent claudication, but no drug has been demonstrated to have analgesic benefit for this type of pain in a double-blind, placebo-controlled, randomized clinical trial. As a consequence, surgical decompression has remained a mainstay of therapy despite lack of consensus about clinical indications and wide geographic variation in rates of surgery [4,5]. There is an even greater evidence gap about the indications for and efficacy of nonsurgical treatments, which likely accounts for even wider variation in their use.

This article aims to characterize the growing unmet need for the treatment of neurogenic intermittent claudication in the elderly population with lumbar spinal stenosis and reviews the current understanding of this

* Corresponding author.
E-mail address: john_markman@urmc.rochester.edu (J.D. Markman).

condition with an eye toward framing a research agenda for nonsurgical treatments.

Background and epidemiology

In his 1954 landmark paper, the Dutch surgeon Verbiest linked progressively worsening leg pain and impairment of motor function experienced upon standing and walking with a narrowed spinal canal [6]. Until he demonstrated that lower extremity claudication could be alleviated with resection of the spinal laminae, such a lower extremity symptom pattern most often was presumed to be caused by peripheral vascular disease involving the aorto–iliac system [7]. The age of symptom onset in the patients in Verbiest's initial series of seven patients, ranging between 37 and 67 years, was far younger than the vast majority of patients who experience symptoms associated with lumbar spinal stenosis today. At that time, life expectancy in the US was 68.2 years [8]. Recent studies reveal an accelerating demographic shift, with most patients seeking treatment for symptomatic lumbar spinal stenosis over the age of 60 at the time of diagnosis [9].

The growing burden of this problem in an aging population is reflected by the fact that approximately 1.2 million physician office visits in the United States are related to symptoms of lumbar spinal stenosis [10]. Pain, neurogenic intermittent claudication in particular, is the predominant symptom pattern prompting treatment [4]. For this chronic pain problem, approximately 125,000 laminectomy procedures were performed in the United States in 1995 [11]. The prevalence of degenerative lumbar spinal stenosis and associated cost are expected to surge as the number of persons aged 60 years or older quadruples to approximately 2 billion worldwide in the year 2050 [12].

Increasing life expectancy will translate into a rapid rise in the number of patient visits for recurrent symptoms of neurogenic claudication in the years following initial surgical treatment [13]. The waning analgesic benefit of lumbar laminectomy over time, and inferior outcomes for patients undergoing repeat decompression will propel this trend [13,14]. Based on 2007 estimated life expectancy, approximately one third of patients who undergo laminectomy may expect to experience approximately 10 years of recurrent neurogenic claudication after surgery. Extending decompression of the spinal canal with repeat surgery in patients who have recurrent neurogenic intermittent claudication symptoms is a more complex proposition, because advanced age carries greater perioperative risk [15]. The risk is compounded, because subsequent decompressive procedures often require instrumentation to prevent the long-term sequelae of spinal instability [16,17].

The rapidly growing population of patients for whom the risk of surgery may outweigh the benefit underscores the need for the development of noninvasive therapies. Among the populations with lumbar spinal stenosis, the elderly stand to benefit the most from an enhanced evidence base about the efficacy of analgesics currently in use and the development of novel, noninvasive therapies. The cost to society of untreated neurogenic claudication is substantial, as older patients who have impaired mobility are less likely to live independently, and reduced activity tolerance further exacerbates the many comorbid conditions that affect elderly patients, such as obesity and diabetes [18].

Pathoanatomy and the limitations of imaging

Non-neural pathoanatomy

Spinal stenosis has been defined as a narrowing of the spinal canal, caused by degeneration of bony and intraspinal soft tissues [19]. The confluence of disc degeneration, facet joint capsule hypertrophy, infolding of the ligamentum flavum, and osteophyte formation culminates in a reduction in the volume of the spinal canal in the degenerative form of lumbar spinal stenosis [20]. Spinal stenosis broadly refers to any site of narrowing in the central canal, lateral recess, or intervertebral foramen. In the elderly, these subtypes frequently coexist [21]. The earliest descriptions of lumbar stenosis focused on developmental forms such as those found in children who had dysrhaphic abnormalities and skeletal dysplasias [22]. Such conditions are beyond the scope of this article, but it is important to note that older patients who have congenitally narrow canals, thickened laminae, and short pedicles are predisposed to the acquired forms of stenosis and often seek medical care for neurogenic intermittent claudication at an earlier age. This article focuses on acquired forms of stenosis. Age-related degeneration of spinal structures associated with the upright posture required for bipedal movement is, by far, the most common form of acquired stenosis.

The progressive collapse of the lumbar disc with normal aging drives segmental narrowing of the lateral recess and central canal. Age-related desiccation of the nucleus pulposus and resultant buckling of the dorsal annulus are most pronounced at the L3 through L5 spinal levels. Not surprisingly, these are the very levels where spinal stenosis is detected most commonly [23]. Loss of disc competency increases biomechanical stress on the facet joints. The resultant hypertrophy of these joints because of synovial overgrowth and subchondral bone formation encroaches on the lateral aspect of the central canal. Progressive change in the orientation and shape of these joints endows the canal with the classic trefoil form seen in the most severe cases. The loss of disc height also decreases tension on the elastic ligamentum flavum that causes buckling of the ligament. Diverse underlying disease processes have been implicated in the development of acquired lumbar stenosis affecting the elderly. These conditions include Paget's disease, rheumatoid arthritis, and bone infiltration by tumors such as prostatic carcinoma. The movement of one anatomic lumbar segment in relation to adjacent levels in the context of degenerative spondylolisthesis is another important cause [24].

The clinical significance of anatomic narrowing is critically related to posture in patients who have lumbar spinal stenosis. Forward flexion increases the cross-sectional area of the neural foramen by 12%. Lumbar extension narrows the canal and lateral recesses by an additional 15% over a neutral posture [25]. Eighty percent of the population have degenerative changes in the spine evident on imaging studies, but most remain asymptomatic [9,26]. The search for a critical threshold of narrowing that separates mild from moderate-to-severe symptoms is complicated by multiple factors other than posture, such as the number of stenotic levels and effects of recurrent dynamic loading, which appear to influence the intensity of pain and degree of activity limitation [27]. Recognition of the lack of sensitivity and specificity of static images has engendered the development of functional concepts of potential space such as spinal reserve capacity [28].

The preeminence of surgical treatments that address canal stenosis has placed a premium on continuous refinement of anatomic measurement. The increasing precision of imaging technology has aided in identifying patients who may benefit most from resection of boney and soft tissue. The concept of the transverse area of the dural sac has supplanted measurement of the anteroposterior diameter championed by Verbiest during the era of myelography. In that era, a distance of less than 10 mm was equated with absolute stenosis [29]. More recently, the measurement of transverse area of the dural sac gained prominence based on retrospective studies of laminectomy patients and in vitro studies of cadaver models [30]. A recent study demonstrated a strong association between the minimum cross-sectional area and walking tolerance in patients undergoing lumbar laminectomy [31]. The borderline minimum canal area between moderate and severe symptoms (eg, inability to walk 500 m or more) consistently has been shown in animal models and retrospective series to be in the 70 mm^2 range. Lateral recess and neuroforaminal stenosis giving rise to unilateral symptom patterns have undergone far less systematic study; an anteroposterior dimension of less than 4 mm in the lateral recess is a threshold frequently cited as a critical level by experts [32].

Neurovascular pathoanatomy

There are characteristic vascular and neuropathologic changes associated with lumbar spinal stenosis and neurogenic intermittent claudication. MRI often reveals dilation of the epidural venous plexus in vivo [33]. Cadaveric studies find constriction of the nerve roots and hypertrophy of the pia-arachnoid [34]. Watanabe detailed a characteristic reduction in number, collapse, and grossly visible congestion of veins proximal to the stenotic level. Histologic and scanning electron microscopy nerve root sections demonstrate a pronounced loss in the count of large-caliber fibers, empty axons, and varying degrees of demyelination. Non-neural changes from these sections included pia-arachnoid adhesions, interstitial fibrosis, and thick-walled veins. Lastly, arteriovenous anastomoses are present. The clinical significance of the adhesive pia-arachnoiditis is unknown, but many have speculated that impedance of normal cerebrospinal fluid (CSF) flow figures prominently in the episodic pain symptoms of neurogenic intermittent claudication.

Recent lines of evidence from animal models indicate that the demyelination and axonal loss in the type of cauda equina injury observed in neurogenic intermittent claudication do not cause mechanical allodynia and hyperalgesia [35]. Those neurologic examination findings are the clinical hallmarks of neuropathic pain classic syndromes such as postherpetic neuralgia (PHN). The absence of these findings likely reflects the relative sparing of the dorsal root ganglion in this type of cauda equina injury and dysfunction, but does not make a neuropathic pain mechanism less likely. The painful symptoms of mild-to-moderate neurogenic intermittent claudication appear to be caused by endoneurial edema produced by mild levels of ischemia [36]. Only the cases of stenosis with severe cauda equina compression will reveal a pathoanatomic finding of wallerian degeneration [37].

In general, less is known about the clinical significance of the vascular and neural changes listed previously, because these structures have not, to date, been the targets of therapeutic intervention. The neuroanatomic changes identified previously have been linked to the chronic inflammatory consequences of episodic neuroischemia presented in the next section.

Pathophysiology of neurogenic intermittent claudication

The underlying pain mechanism of the unique symptom pattern known as neurogenic intermittent claudication is a matter of controversy. Narrowing of the spinal canal simply does not equate to pain. A compelling account of the pathophysiology must at once account for the many patients with stenosis who experience no pain and the large population whose pain is relieved effectively with anatomic decompression [26]. Increases in pressure applied to the cauda equina induce neurophysiologic and local hemodynamic changes. The lines of experimental evidence and in vivo clinical observations point to an underlying neurovascular mechanism [38,39]. The intricate relationship between recurrent inadequate blood flow, compromised metabolic status of the nerve roots, modulating inflammatory cell effects on the blood–nerve barrier, and the pain of neurogenic intermittent claudication is in need of further study. There is convincing evidence that both the lesions of the nervous system discussed previously and the dysfunction of the cauda equina reviewed in this section are linked tightly to the experience of pain in patients who experience neurogenic intermittent claudication. Viewed in this way, neurogenic intermittent claudication represents a neuropathic pain syndrome with a distinctive localization and clinical phenomenology.

Beyond mechanical compression

Intermittent direct mechanical compression of the cauda equina by osseous and soft tissues was the leading putative cause of neurogenic intermittent claudication and other neurologic deficits in lumbar spinal stenosis for much of the last century. Such an explanation provided the rationale for laminectomy in the 1950s. There are several features of the clinical syndrome that are not typical of neural entrapment syndromes:

1. The rapidity of symptom relief with change of posture;
2. The absence of sensory and motor signs in many patients who have severe narrowing;
3. The lack of analgesic or functional benefit in approximately one third of patients who have neurogenic claudication undergoing extensive surgical decompression.

Although direct mechanical compression of neural structures may cause symptoms in a subpopulation of patients with the most severely narrowed canals, it does not account for the episodic pain experienced by the vast majority of patients with symptoms that rapidly remit with postural adjustment.

Animal models and in vivo studies have correlated neurogenic intermittent claudication with increases in intraspinal pressure. Lumbar epidural pressure is elevated (peak values are 82.8 mm Hg) when the volume of the canal is reduced, most commonly with walking and prolonged standing in an erect posture [40]. The direct relationship between intraspinal pressure and extensor postures is the best-understood aspect of the syndrome's pathophysiology; it has been quantified with manometry and directly observed with myeloscopy in symptomatic patients [41]. Increased pressure and venous engorgement, much like the boney changes, are not likely the proximal cause of pain, because both of these phenomena are observed commonly in asymptomatic patients who have radiographic evidence of stenosis. The predictability with which pressure changes normalize with postural adjustment (eg, flexion) and alleviate pain symptoms, however, underscores the clinical significance of this association.

Microcirculatory derangement

Multiple lines of evidence point to the importance of diminished flow of CSF, arterial, and venous blood in the pathophysiology of neurogenic intermittent claudication [42]. Elevated intraspinal pressures reduce the flow of CSF. Up to 58% of nerve root tissue nutrients are supplied by the CSF in porcine models [43]. The relatively thin epineurium and perineurium of the nerve roots with their fenestrated outer layers facilitate this source of nutrition. Cauda equina metabolism, not unlike a tract in the central nervous system, is critically dependent on CSF flow. It has been proposed that hypertrophic thickening of the pia-arachnoid is the sine qua non of claudication etiology [34]. An adhesive pia-arachnoiditis at the most stenotic levels likely impairs diffusion of CSF. This reduced permeability, coupled with compromised CSF flow, may provoke a localized hypometabolic state in the nerve root(s) at symptomatic levels. The cumulative nature of these changes might explain why there appears to be a prolonged asymptomatic phase lasting years in patients who have lumbar stenosis. A prolonged course of episodic inflammation may be required to induce a symptomatic proliferation of connective tissue in the pia-arachnoid.

Arnoldi and others have advocated that increased venous congestion underpins the pain of neurogenic claudication [44]. He assumed the relatively thin walls of venous structures are more vulnerable to the mechanical stress of elevated intraspinal pressure. Olmarker has shown that increased mechanical pressure in pigs could cause disturbances in the blood supply and the nutrition of the nerve roots; he characterized the direct relationship between increased pressure and impairment of nerve conduction [45,46]. A 10 mm Hg change in pressure was sufficient to induce occlusion in some venules, and a 64% reduction in total blood flow [47,48]. Microvascular arterial insufficiency of the nerve roots has been invoked to explain the spectrum of reversible symptoms in neurogenic intermittent claudication. The major weakness of the arterial hypothesis, and to a lesser extent the venous story, is that the natural history of lumbar stenosis is not associated with infarcts of the roots or cauda equina, and fixed deficits (eg, weakness) are rare [49].

Endothelial dysfunction that alters neural metabolism of the cauda equina may offer a more compelling account of what is observed clinically in patients who have a syndrome of neurogenic intermittent claudication that does not culminate with infarction. An experimental constriction injury model in adult dogs evaluated breakdown of the blood–nerve barrier. In this study, intraradicular edema was detected with gadolinium-enhanced imaging [50]. Nerve root macrophage invasion associated with increased vascular permeability appears to provoke an inflammatory neuritis [51]. Macrophage generation of interleukin (IL)-1, tumor necrosis factor (TNF), and other mediators of the inflammatory process likely play a role in the pathogenesis of neurogenic intermittent claudication [35].

Nerve conduction properties in porcine models are altered by intermittent compression of the cauda equine [52]. These neurophysiologic changes are homologous to the F wave prolongation recorded in people who have symptoms of neurogenic intermittent claudication [53]. Animal models of chronic pain of this type in bipedal primates are not available. The activation of extracellular signal-regulated protein kinase (ERK) in superficial dorsal horn neurons appears to correlate with reduced running tolerance in a rat model of neurogenic intermittent claudication [54]. A prostaglandin E1 analog improves walking dysfunction in this model. The improvement is associated with reduced phosphorylation of ERK and attenuated decrease in spinal cord blood flow due to vasodilation [55]. This pathway offers one possible target for novel pharmacotherapy.

Natural history of lumbar spinal stenosis

The onset of neurogenic claudication in the setting of lumbar stenosis is insidious and commonly heralded by a long history of central low back pain

[56]. A recent longitudinal, prospective, controlled cohort study of patients who chose not to undergo decompressive surgery upheld the claim that lumbar spinal stenosis is not associated with progressive neurologic deficit [57]. The authors found that the natural history of lumbar stenosis is characterized by fluctuation in symptom severity and a tendency toward modest improvement in patients who do not elect to undergo surgery. In his landmark study, Johnsson compared the course of 19 untreated patients who had myelographically-defined, lumbar spinal stenosis for a mean of 4 years. Eighty percent of these patients experienced neurogenic intermittent claudication. Severe neurologic deterioration was not found in the untreated patients; approximately 60% of these patients were unchanged from the standpoint of symptom severity [58].

The prospective, long-term observational studies by Amundsen and colleagues [59] and the Maine Lumbar Spine Study offer valuable insights about the natural history of this condition. At 4 years, the Amundsen study found superior outcomes in a greater number of surgically treated patients, but results of delayed surgery in the patients in the conservative management group who crossed over were comparable. In Atlas' study at 8- to 10-year follow-up, low back pain relief, predominant symptom improvement, and current symptoms did not differ for those initially receiving conservative or surgical treatment. Leg pain relief and function as measured by the modified Roland disability scale favored those managed surgically at the outset. In summary, the syndrome of lumbar spinal stenosis is marked by periodic exacerbations and remittances [60].

Diagnosis

Increased use of axial imaging has led to a sharp increase in the diagnosis of lumbar spinal stenosis, but these technologies do not differentiate symptomatic from asymptomatic patients. For this reason, it is essential to obtain a thorough history, perform a neurologic examination, conduct functional testing, and place anatomic imaging results in the clinical context. Advanced age, severe lower extremity pain, and absence of pain when seated are the historical findings most strongly associated (likelihood ratio of at least 2) with the diagnosis of lumbar spinal stenosis in a group of 93 patients from three different specialty clinics [56]. Physical examination findings most consistent with the diagnosis were wide-based gait, abnormal Romberg test result, thigh pain following 30 seconds of lumbar extension, and neuromuscular deficits. The quality of the pain is classically dull or aching and characterized as heaviness or weakness.

Because degenerative changes in multiple spinal structures are ubiquitous in the elderly, the primary role of imaging in this population with chronic symptoms is in the planning of surgical intervention. Imaging obtained in the supine position may underestimate narrowing that would be apparent in an upright, weight-bearing position [61]. Imaging acute, nonspecific low back pain has been shown to yield many diagnoses of lumbar spinal stenosis with little clinical relevance [62]. If narrowing of the canal is observed, and surgery is considered, CT combined with myelography (CTM) will provide the most sensitive picture of posture-dependent anatomic targets. In CTM, myelography is performed first with the patient in flexed and extended standing positions. The myelogram is an invasive technique that allows visualization of boney and soft tissue encroachment on the dural sac in the symptomatic posture [63].

Because the degree of narrowing observed in imaging often does not correlate to the severity of symptoms, functional testing should complement imaging. Treadmill testing has been shown to be a safe, easy, and reliable method of assessing a patient's response to treatment [64,65]. The unique clinical phenomenology of neurogenic claudication lends itself to objective measure because of its direct impact on the amount of time patients are able to stand and the distance they are able to walk. The value of an endpoint that links pain intensity and function is clear to the patient timing his or her medication dose to enable a walk to the post office box or trip down a grocery aisle. The capacity to assess dose-dependent responses to therapy over time is also critical to the task of adapting treadmill-based methodologies to the evaluation of novel therapeutic strategies. The incorporation of regular treadmill testing will allow for more precise treatment matching for surgical therapies and ultimately guide dose titration of emerging therapeutics. Electromyogram (EMG) mapping of the lumbar paraspinal musculature has been advocated by some experts as a superior tool to MRI to differentiate symptomatic from asymptomatic patients with lumbar spinal stenosis [66].

Differential diagnosis

Although neurogenic intermittent claudication associated with lumbar spinal stenosis is a common condition, other etiologies may create a similar symptom pattern, especially in the elderly, where patients may have multiple comorbid conditions. Back and leg pain, numbness and paresthesias are common symptoms associated with lumbar spinal stenosis. A thorough investigation for nondegenerative causes of pain must be undertaken to address possibilities such as a tumor, infection, and vascular causes in circumstances where risk factors or so-called red flags are present. These are rare causes of spinal pain, but they may be life-threatening. History taking and physical examination should exclude aortic aneurysm, visceral diseases such as pyelonephritis, and systemic inflammatory conditions including polymyalgia rheumatica. The differential diagnosis includes vascular claudication, which will not be affected by posture, and is less likely if peripheral pulses are palpable. Vascular claudication can coexist with neurogenic intermittent claudication and should be ruled out with flow studies if there is clinical suspicion.

In most cases, the diagnostic challenge resides in parsing the low back and leg pain of lumbar stenosis from other mechanical causes of pain localizing to soft tissues, joints, and boney sources. Herniated lumbar disk with corresponding level radiculitis and peripheral neuropathy are common considerations. A herniated lumbar disk typically has a distinctive temporal pattern marked by acute onset of symptoms and other examination features such as pain elicited with straight leg raise testing. Inflammation associated with facet-mediated pain causes axial predominant symptoms. Because postures such as standing and walking require lumbar extension that load the facet joint, symptoms of this type of mechanical syndrome can overlap with lumbar spinal stenosis or mimic the distribution and pattern of symptom provocation. Osteoporotic compression fractures have a distinctive pattern of symptom onset (ie, rapid), commonly provoke pain in the seated and supine position, and have a distinctive set of findings on imaging. Neurogenic intermittent claudication and osteoporotic compression fractures may coexist when there is concurrent stenosis at the symptomatic level because of associated change in canal dimensions. Electrophysiological techniques such as the tibial F-wave can be useful in distinguishing between lumbar spinal stenosis and peripheral neuropathy in cases where multiple neuropathic syndromes are thought to coexist. The key distinguishing feature of lumbar stenosis is neurogenic intermittent claudication. Case reports of pain provoked by extension and exertion that remits with rest have been reported in cases of tumors of the conus medullaris and cauda equina, benign cystic lesions, and vascular malformations, but these instances are exceptional).

Treatment

Treatment approaches for lumbar stenosis target the low back and leg pain localizing to the cauda equina with the distinctive phenomenology of neurogenic intermittent claudication. Increasing activity interference with standing and walking and escalating pain intensity compel patients to seek treatment. The decision to pursue treatment for a fluctuating symptom pattern is highly personalized. Change in societal beliefs about the experience of pain, expectations for function, and the goal of independent living beyond the seventh decade of life appear to be driving increased use of all treatments for chronic low back pain [67]. Increased reliance on diagnostic imaging by providers is another powerful driver of surging demand for treatment [68].

There is wide variation in the rates of use of different treatment methods. The preponderance of evidence related to outcomes of lumbar spinal stenosis treatment is found in the surgical literature focusing on decompressive laminectomy. There is a relatively robust evidence base supporting the efficacy of laminectomy, but there is significant uncertainty about optimal timing, the advantages of newer techniques and technologies, the durability of functional improvement, and the benefit of surgery compared with nonsurgical approaches. There is a major gap in the evidence base with respect to the controlled evaluation of conservative management [69,70].

Nonsurgical approaches

In elderly patients at risk for perioperative complications and in those who have mild-to-moderate symptom severity, surgery is often not the preferred treatment [21,71]. For these groups of patients and the substantial number of patients who have neurogenic claudication that recurs after surgery, conservative treatment may be more appropriate [59,72]. Because the symptom of lumbar spinal stenosis is provoked by specific activities, the most common intervention is activity modification. Many patients control their experience of pain by simply curtailing time spent standing or the distances walked. The other ubiquitous patient-initiated strategy to control pain is forward flexion at the lumbar spine. Patients experiencing neurogenic intermittent claudication often unconsciously modify their posture to reduce symptoms; others classically report extended walking tolerance when adapting to an activity such as when leaning on a shopping cart. The use of a walker or walking stick promotes this postural adjustment; these appliances are likely the most common solution for neurogenic intermittent claudication. As with other treatment approaches, patient treatment preference is of paramount importance, because even the most advanced cases of lumbar spinal stenosis rarely are associated with irreversible neurologic deficit. It is critical to remember that such reversibility is not true of stenosis at the cervical and thoracic levels where the spinal cord may be compressed. At these spinal levels, surgical decompression frequently spares permanent neurologic deficit and represents definitive treatment.

Studies of nonoperative treatment for lumbar spinal stenosis invariably advocate for exercise regimens that include strengthening, general stretching, McKenzie method of passive end-range stretching exercises, and conventional physical therapy. Although there is evidence that exercise appears to increase the rate of return to normal activities in patients who have persistent low back pain, virtually none of these studies focus on the syndrome of lumbar spinal stenosis or the symptom pattern of neurogenic intermittent claudication [73]. Exercises that strengthen the abdominal core muscles and promote mobility of the lumbar paraspinal muscles may offer benefit, because they can stabilize the lumbar spine and minimize lordosis [74]. Cardiovascular conditioning can be beneficial by promoting weight loss, as heavier patients may be more likely to develop the degenerative changes leading to stenosis [75]. Multiple studies of conservative, or nonoperative treatment, with various physical therapy approaches have found that most (approximately 70%) of patients perceived no worsening of their symptoms and a smaller number (approximately 15%) reported improvement [72]. In Simotas' study, the surgical groups tended to report greater reduction in leg pain intensity and improved activity tolerance, but approximately 30% of conservatively managed patients in one cohort study reported no pain or minimal pain at 36 months.

There is scant evidence supporting the use of oral analgesics for the symptom pattern of neurogenic intermittent claudication. The only positive drug trial specifically targeting this condition is a recent, unblinded randomized trial of gabapentin. Gabapentin is an amino acid thought to modulate pain intensity through interaction with an axillary subunit of voltage-dependent Ca^{++} channels [76]. In this study, 55 patients were randomized to conservative management with corset and nonsteroidal anti-inflammatory drugs (NSAIDs) or gabapentin (maximum 2400 mg) in addition to conservative therapy over 4 months. The patients in the gabapentin group demonstrated a statistically significant increase in walking distance and a decrease in the intensity of low back and leg pain (Visual Analogue Scale) upon movement. The favorable results of this trial should be interpreted with caution because of the enhanced placebo effect expected with lack of blinding.

Promising early results for the treatment of Paget's disease prompted a trial of calcitonin for neurogenic claudication. Porter reported 11 patients who had improved walking tolerance associated with calcitonin 100 U administered four times per week for four weeks [77]. This polypeptide hormone secreted by the para-follicular cells of the thyroid was thought to possess both analgesic and anti-inflammatory properties in addition to the promotion of osteoclastic bone resorption that accounts for efficacy in Paget's disease. A large well-designed double-bind, randomized, placebo-controlled trial of a nasal spray formulation failed to show improvement in pain or walking time to first pain. Other, nonrandomized studies have reported an improvement in pain scores, but in a second randomized, well-designed study, the benefit compared with placebo did not reach statistical significance [78].

Anti-inflammatory therapy with NSAIDs and more selective cyclooxygenase-2 inhibitors have analgesic benefit compared with placebo in the minimally detectable range for chronic low back pain [79]. There were no trials available to be included in this meta-analysis designed to assess patients who had neurogenic intermittent claudication. Recent evidence of increased cardiovascular risk with long-term use of these medication classes in higher-risk individuals renders this group of agents a less appealing option from a risk–benefit perspective [80]. There is evidence supporting the use of opioids for chronic low back pain [72], but their analgesic benefit in neurogenic intermittent claudication remains unknown. In general, opioids appear to be less effective for movement-evoked pain.

Lumbar epidural steroid injections are used commonly for treating neurogenic intermittent claudication in lumbar spinal stenosis despite controversy about their role [81,82]. The rationale for this treatment is reduction of the intraradicular edema and inflammatory cell infiltration associated with the pain of neurogenic intermittent claudication [50]. There are no prospective, placebo-controlled studies evaluating the use of epidural steroid injection specifically for spinal stenosis. This therapy often is considered a second-tier conservative approach to managing neurogenic intermittent claudication in patients who wish to avoid surgery. Delport and colleagues [83] described the outcomes of epidural steroid injection in a retrospective review of 140 patients. She and her colleagues found that among patients receiving epidural corticosteroid injections, one third experienced relief for greater than 2 months, and more than 50% of patients demonstrated an improvement in walking tolerance. One recent study was unable to determine the critical spinal canal dimensions, as measured by CT scanning, which would be more predictive of a response to interlaminar epidural steroid injection [84]. A second retrospective study showed reduction in pain intensity that correlated with the number of stenotic levels and degree of stenosis except in patients who had greater than three levels and MRI findings rated as severe [85].

Surgical approaches

Since its original conception as a disease caused by boney anatomic changes, clinical study of lumbar stenosis has emphasized surgical treatment. Decompressive laminectomy aims to afford pain relief, improve mobility, preserve neural tissue, and prevent worsening of clinical deficits if present. There are multiple surgical techniques ranging from multilevel decompressive laminectomies, unilateral decompressive hemilaminectomy, and multilevel laminotomy with a fenestrating technique that preserves the interspinous ligaments in widespread use. The technique typically involves excision of the ligamentum flavum and partial removal of the laminae; medial facetectomies and foraminotomies often are performed also. Surgical treatment is considered to be the most effective treatment modality in patients who have symptomatic lumbar stenosis and neurogenic intermittent claudication [4].

Turner's attempted meta-analysis in 1991, which included 74 studies of laminectomy, found good-to-excellent outcomes at long-term follow-up of 64%. The rates of successful surgical outcomes vary widely [4,86]. The authors' critique of the surgical literature described heterogeneity with regard to patient population, patient selection, and outcome measures. Since that time, several prospective, long-term, observational follow-up studies attempting to evaluate conservative versus surgical treatment have been completed. Surgery repeatedly has been shown to improve short-term outcomes, but long-term outcomes are less favorable as compared with other approaches [14,87]. The Maine lumbar spine study found that for patients who have persistent radicular leg pain, radiologic signs of stenosis, nerve root compression, and no previous back surgery, outcomes are superior with surgery than with conservative care [13]. The consensus emerging from this body of research is that deferring surgical intervention does not preclude a favorable outcome at a later date.

A recent cohort study of long-term outcome of laminectomy in octogenarians (average age at time of surgery 82.2 years) with follow-up at 1.5 years resulted in an improvement in back-related functional status (Oswestry Disability Index) consistent with results in younger age groups, reduction in pain intensity, and use of opioid and NSAIDs [17]. The authors cited the low complication rate in this small group (ie, perioperative delirium in three patients and persistent bladder dysfunction in one patient) as evidence of the safety of this procedure in older patents. Despite the improvement in pain and function, however, only 65% of patients endorsed general satisfaction with their surgery. The authors hypothesized that this finding may be attributed to concurrent depression in 5 of the 23 patients in this study.

Depression has a relatively high prevalence (36% in one cohort, $n = 3801$) in patients who have lumbar spinal stenosis, and it has been associated with higher pain intensity, worsened functional status, and poorer surgical outcomes [88]. The most common cause of failure of this procedure is poor selection of patients; however, clear data on which patients are the best candidates for this surgery are lacking [86,89]. Coexisting cardiovascular morbidity and scoliosis also predict poorer patient rating of outcome, whereas better baseline walking ability, higher self-rated health, higher income, reduced coexisting disease, and pronounced central stenosis predict a more favorable outcome [90].

Surgical indications must be considered carefully, especially in elderly patients, who often have many comorbid conditions placing them at risk for perioperative complications and less favorable outcome in certain circumstances. Patients should be counseled that the likelihood of benefit from laminectomy likely will be limited in the case of multilevel stenosis; functional gains also may be reduced in the context of a coexisting musculoskeletal disorder. One commonly cited liability specific to laminectomy is compromise of the structure of the lumbar motion segment that in turn may lead to further degeneration, excessive or abnormal motion, or deformity. Lumbar fusion was thought to have the benefit of providing definitive stabilization along with decompression. Since the introduction of new fusion technologies, the Washington State registry has seen a 32% greater likelihood of reoperation after the first year postoperatively following an initial fusion, compared with decompression alone for the indication of lumbar spinal stenosis [91]. Microdecompression is a less invasive method of decompression designed to minimize this iatrogenic insult [92]. Patient satisfaction with microdecompression has been high, but it is a procedure in which success requires great technical skill and surgical experience. Evidence on the relative benefit of this approach compared with conventional laminectomy is limited. Because of the risk of early failure, recurrence of symptoms, and complications, a shared decision-making model is essential when considering treatment with laminectomy for patients who have persistent, moderate-to-severe neurogenic intermittent claudication.

Interspinous process spacers are a new class of implantable devices that recently received US Food and Drug Administration (FDA) approval. This device creates a relative kyphosis at the level of insertion, reducing extension while allowing flexion [93]. Various designs, ranging from static spacers to dynamic (ie, spring like), are inserted surgically between adjacent spinous processes at the culprit level. This type of approach first was introduced in the 1950s but fell out of favor because of a tendency to become displaced over time [94].

The first approved device in this class, the X STOP (St. Francis Medical Technologies, Concord, California), has an indication for mild-to-moderate neurogenic intermittent claudication on the basis of a multicenter, prospective, randomized trial with 191 patients [95]. Many features of the study design and the use of the neurogenic intermittent claudication as an endpoint represent important advances in the evaluation of treatments for lumbar spinal stenosis. The device was compared with nonoperative treatment, and the primary endpoint was a questionnaire designed to assess symptom severity and physical function domains related to neurogenic intermittent claudication. At 2 years, there was a significant improvement in symptoms and function as compared with epidural steroid injection and conservative therapy. One important limitation is the use of a single epidural steroid injection in most patients as a comparator when the half-life of the injected anti-inflammatory medication is on the order of weeks. The authors compared the outcomes of the X STOP placement to Katz's study of laminectomy but highlighted the higher risk of complication for laminectomy (12.6% from the Turner meta-analysis) in contrast with the relative absence of complications from the superficial placement of the new device.

Interspinous process spacers require smaller exposure, local anesthesia, and less time than laminectomy. The challenge of identifying the culprit level of stenosis that correlates with symptoms is more crucial than ever, because there is not the flexibility to extend resection as in the case of laminectomy. Placement of such devices may prove to be a safer option for elderly patients than the traditional, more invasive procedures, but longer-term follow-up is needed.

Future considerations

There is a rapidly growing, unmet clinical need for nonsurgical therapies for neurogenic intermittent claudication, the primary symptom of lumbar spinal stenosis for which patients seek treatment. Neurogenic intermittent claudication is an episodic neuropathic pain syndrome localizing to the cauda equina. Animal models have revealed key insights into the underlying pain mechanisms of neurogenic intermittent claudication and validated a host of therapeutic targets for medical treatment. With the adaptation of treadmill-based clinical trial methodologies developed to assess surgical outcomes, there is a foundation for better treatment matching for common surgical procedures and compelling endpoints to assess the efficacy of novel therapies. The regulatory pathway for therapies targeting neurogenic intermittent claudication has been opened with the recent approval of a novel class of spinal devices. A new generation of nonsurgical therapies for treating lumbar spinal stenosis and neurogenic intermittent claudication will offer the possibility of improved mobility and independence throughout the lifespan.

Summary

- Lumbar spinal stenosis is a leading cause of impaired mobility in the geriatric population.
- Neurogenic intermittent claudication is the principal painful symptom pattern for which patients seek treatment.
- Laminectomy remains a mainstay of therapy, but there is wide variation in rates of surgery and outcomes that may reflect an overemphasis on pathoanatomy driven by over-reliance on imaging technology.
- Recent advances in the understanding of the pathophysiology of this distinctive neuropathic syndrome localizing to the cauda equina will provide the foundation for nonsurgical therapies for which there is a growing unmet need.

References

[1] Taylor VM, Deyo RA, Cherkin DC, et al. Low back pain hospitalization: recent US trends and regional variations. Spine 1994;19:1207–11.
[2] Weiner DK. Office management of chronic pain in the elderly. Am J Med 2007;120(4): 306–15.
[3] Bennett G. Neuropathic pain: an overview. In: Borsook D, editor. Molecular neurobiology of pain, progress in pain research and management, vol. 9. Seattle (WA): IASP Press; 1997.
[4] Turner JA, Ersek M, Herron L, et al. Surgery for lumbar spinal stenosis: attempted meta-analysis of the literature. Spine 1992;17(1):1–8.
[5] Deyo RA, Mirza SK. Trends and variations in the use of spine surgery. Clin Orthop Relat Res 2006;443:139–46.
[6] Verbiest H. A radicular syndrome from developmental narrowing of the lumbar vertebral canal. J Bone Joint Surg Br 1954;36(2):230–7.
[7] Sugar O. Jean-Francois Bouley. Spine 1994;19:346–9.
[8] National Center for Health Statistics. Health, United States, 2006: with chartbook on trends in the health of Americans. US Dept of Health and Human Services, Centers for Disease Control and Prevention. Hyattsville (MD); 2006.
[9] Kauffman C, Garfin SR. Spinal stenosis: pathophysiology and symptom complex update 1999. Semin Spine Surg 1999;11(3):209–14.
[10] Hart LG, Deyo RA, Cherkin DC. Physician office visits for low back pain. Frequency, clinical evaluation, and treatment patterns from a U.S. national survey. Spine 1995;20:11–9.
[11] The Ortho FactBook (TM): U.S. 5th edition. Knowledge Enterprises, Inc; Chagrin Falls, Ohio 2005. Solucient, LLC and Verispan, LLC.
[12] U.S. Kinsella K. and Velkoff VA. An Aging World: 2001. International Population Reports. US Department of Health and Human Services, US Department of Commerce, 2002;23–47.

[13] Atlas SJ, Keller RB, Wu YA, et al. Long-term outcomes of surgical and nonsurgical management of lumbar spinal stenosis: 8- to 10-year results from the Maine lumbar spine study.
Spine 2005;30(8):936–43.

[14] Postacchini F. Spine update: surgical management of lumbar stenosis. Spine 1999;24(10):
1043–7.

[15] Katz JN, Stucki G, Lipson SJ, et al. Predictors of surgical outcome in degenerative lumbar
spinal stenosis. Spine 1999;24:2229–33.

[16] Deyo RA, Ciol MA, Cherkin DC, et al. Lumbar spine fusion: a cohort study of complications, reoperations, and resource use of the Medicare population. Spine 1993;18:1463–70.

[17] Galiano K, Obwegeser AA, Gabl MV, et al. Long-term outcome of laminectomy for spinal
stenosis in octogenarians. Spine 2005;30(3):332–5.

[18] Loureiroa ML, Nayga RM. Obesity, weight loss, and physician's advice. Soc Sci Med 2006;
62(10):2458–68.

[19] Porter RW. Spinal stenosis and neurogenic claudication. Spine 1996;21:2046–52.

[20] Andersson GB. Surgical aspects on lateral spinal stenosis: indications and principles. Acta
Orthopaedica Scandinavica Supplementum (Suppl 251) 1993;64:74–5.

[21] Onel D, Hidayet S, Cigdem D. Lumbar spinal stenosis: clinical/radiologic therapeutic
evaluation in 145 patients. Spine 1993;18:291–8.

[22] Binder DK, Schmidt MH, Weinstein PR. Lumbar spinal stenosis. Semin Neurol 2002;22(2):
157–65.

[23] Lewin T. Osteoarthritis in lumbar synovial joints. A morphologic study. Acta Orthop Scand
Suppl 1964;73:1–112.

[24] Akuthota V, Lento P, Sowa G. Pathogenesis of lumbar spinal stenosis pain: why does an
asymptomatic stenotic patient flare? Phys Med Rehabil Clin N Am 2003;14:17–28.

[25] Inufusa A, An HS, Lim TH, et al. Anatomic changes of the spinal canal and intervertebral
foramen associated with flexion–extension movement. Spine 1996;21(21):2412–20.

[26] Boden SD, Davis DO, Dina TS, et al. Abnormal magnetic resonance scans of the lumbar
spine in asymptomatic subjects: a prospective investigation. J Bone Joint Surg Am 1990;
72:403–8.

[27] Johnson KE, Rosen I, Uden A. The natural course of lumbar spinal stenosis. Clin Orthop
Relat Res 1992;279:82–6.

[28] Weisz GM, Lee P. Spinal canal stenosis. Clin Orthop Relat Res 1983;178:134–40.

[29] Verbiest H. Neurogenic intermittent claudication in cases with absolute and relative stenosis
of the lumbar vertebral canal (ASLC and RSLC), in cases with narrow lumbar intervertebral
foramina, and in cases with both entities. Clin Neurosurg 1973;20:204–14.

[30] Schonstrom N, Willen J. Imaging lumbar spinal stenosis. Radiol Clin North Am 2001;39:
31–53.

[31] Ogikubo O, Forsberg L, Hanson T. The relationship between the cross-sectional area of the
cauda equina and the preoperative symptom of central lumbar spinal stenosis. Spine 2007;
32:1423–8.

[32] Eisenstein S. Lumbar vertebral canal morphometry for computerized tomography in spinal
stenosis. Spine 1983;8:187–91.

[33] Manaka M, Komagata M, Endo K, et al. Assessment of lumbar spinal canal stenosis by
magnetic resonance phlebography. J Orthop Sci 2003;8:1–7.

[34] Watanabe R, Parke WW. Vascular and neural pathology of lumbosacral spinal stenosis.
J Neurosurg 1986;64:64–70.

[35] Sekiguchi M, Kikuchi S, Myers RR. Experimental spinal stenosis. Spine 2004;29(10):
1105–11.

[36] Sekiguchi M, Konno S, Anzai H, et al. Nerve vasculature changes induced by serotonin
under chronic cauda equina compression. Spine 2002;27:1634–9.

[37] Powell HC, Myers RR. Pathology of experimental nerve compression. Lab Invest 1986;139:
28–38.

[38] Blau JN, Logue V. Intermittent claudication of the cauda equina: an unusual syndrome resulting from central protrusion of a lumbar intervertebral disc. Lancet 1961;1:1081–6.

[39] Rydevik B, Brown M, Lundborg G. Pathoanatomy and pathophysiology of nerve root compression. Spine 1984;9:7–15.

[40] Takahashi K, Kagechika K, Takino T, et al. Changes in epidural pressure during walking in patients with lumbar spinal stenosis. Spine 1995;20:2746–9.

[41] Ooi Y, Mita F, Satoh Y. Myeloscopic study on lumbar spinal canal stenosis with special reference to intermittent claudication. Spine 1990;15(6):544–9.

[42] Rydevik B. Neurophysiology of cauda equina compression. Acta Orthop Scand (Suppl 251) 1993;64:52–5.

[43] Olmarker K, Rydevik B, Hansson T, et al. Compression-induced changes of the nutritional supply to the porcine cauda equine. J Spinal Disord 1990;3:25–9.

[44] Arnoldi CC, Brodsky AE, Cauchoix J, et al. Lumbar spinal stenosis and nerve root entrapment syndromes. Clin Orthop 1976;115:4–5.

[45] Olmarker K, Rydevik B. Single- versus double-level nerve root compression. An experimental study on the porcine cauda equina with analyses of nere impulse conduction properties. Clin Orthop Relat Res 1992;279:35–9.

[46] Olmarker K, Holm S, Rydevik B. Importance of compression onset rate for the degree of impairment of impulse propagation in experimental compression injury of the porcine cauda equine. Spine 1990;15:416–9.

[47] Takahashi K, Olmareker K, Holms S, et al. Double-level cauda equina compression: an experimental study with continuous monitoring of intraneural blood flow in the porcine cauda equina. J Orthop Res 1993;11(1):104–9.

[48] Rydevik BL, Pedowitz RA, Hargens AR, et al. Effects of acute, graded compression on spinal nerve root function and structure: an experimental study of the pig cauda equina. Spine 1991;16(5):487–93.

[49] Parke WW, Watanabe R. The intrinsic vasculature of the lumbosacral spinal nerve roots. Spine 1985;10:508–15.

[50] Kobayashi S, Uchida K, Takeno K, et al. Imaging of cauda equina edema in lumbar canal stenosis by using gadolinium-enhanced MR imaging: experimental constriction injury. AJNR Am J Neuroradiol 2006;27:346–53.

[51] Kobayashi S, Baba H, Uchida K, et al. Localization and changes of intraneural inflammatory cytokines and inducible nitric oxide induced by mechanical compression. J Orthop Res 2005;23:771–8.

[52] Konno S, Olmarker K, Byrod G, et al. Intermittent cauda equina compression: an experimental study on the porcine cauda equina with analyses of nerve impulse conduction properties. Spine 1995;20:1223–6.

[53] London SF, England JD. Dynamic F waves in neurogenic claudication. Muscle Nerve 1991; 14:457–61.

[54] Liu Y, Obata K, Yamanaka H, et al. Activation of extracellular signal-regulated protein kinase in dorsal horn neurons in the rat neuropathic intermittent claudication model. Pain 2004;109:64–72.

[55] Takenobu Y, Katsube N, Marsala M, et al. Model of neuropathic intermittent claudication in the rat: methodology and application. J Neurosci 2001;104:191–8.

[56] Katz JN, Dalgas M, Stucki G, et al. Degenerative lumbar spinal stenosis: diagnostic value of the history and physical examination. Arthritis Rheum 1995;38(9):1236–41.

[57] Haig AJ, Tong HC, Yamakawa KSJ, et al. Predictors of pain and function in persons with spinal stenosis, low back pain, and no back pain. Spine 2006;31(5):2950–7.

[58] Johnsson KE, Uden A, Rosen I. The effect of decompression on the natural course of spinal stenosis: a comparison of surgically treated and untreated patients. Spine 1991;16:615–9.

[59] Amundsen T, Weber H, Nordal H, et al. Lumbar spinal stenosis: conservative or surgical management? A prospective 10-year study. Spine 2000;25(11):1424–36.

[60] Atlas SJ, Keller RB, Robson D, et al. Surgical and nonsurgical management of lumbar spinal stenosis. Four-year outcomes from the Maine lumbar spine study. Spine 2000;25: 556–62.
[61] Saint-Louis LA. Lumbar spinal stenosis assessment with computed tomography, magnetic resonance imaging, and myelography. Clin Orthop Relat Res 2001;384:122–36.
[62] Jinkins JR. MR evaluation of stenosis involving the neural foramina, lateral recesses, and central canal of the lumbosacral spine. Magn Reson Imaging Clin N Am 1999;7(3): 493–511.
[63] Willen J, Danielsson B, Gaulitz A, et al. Dynamic effects on the lumbar spinal canal. Spine 1997;24:2968–76.
[64] Tenhula J, Lenke LG, Bridwell KH, et al. Prospective functional evaluation of the surgical treatment of neurogenic claudication in patients with lumbar spinal stenosis. J Spinal Disord 2000;13(4):276–82.
[65] Deen GH, Zimmerman RS, Lyons MK, et al. Test–retest reproducibility of the exercise treadmill examination in lumbar spinal stenosis. Mayo Clin Proc 2000;75(10):1002–7.
[66] Chiodo A, Haig AJ, Yamakawa KSJ, et al. Needle EMG has a lower false-positive rate than MRI in asymptomatic older adults being evaluated for lumbar spinal stenosis. Clin Neurophysiol 2007;118:751–6.
[67] Friedly J, Chan L, Deyo R. Increases in lumbarosacral injection in the Medicare population. Spine 2007;32(16):1754–60.
[68] Ciol M, Deyo R, Howell E, et al. An assessment of surgery for spinal stenosis: time trends, geographic variations, complications, and reoperations. J Am Geriatr Soc 1996; 44:285–90.
[69] Vogt M, Kwoh C, Cope D, et al. Analgesic usage for low back pain: impact on health care costs and service use. Spine 2005;9:1075–81.
[70] Podichetty V, Segal A, Lieber M, et al. Effectiveness of salmon calcitonin nasal spray in the treatment of lumbar canal stenosis: a double-blind, randomized, placebo-controlled, parallel group trial. Spine 2004;29:2343–9.
[71] Deyo RA. Back surgery—who needs it? N Engl J Med 2007;356(22):2239–43.
[72] Simotas AC, Dorey FJ, Hansraj KK, et al. Nonoperative treatment for lumbar spinal stenosis: clinical and outcome results and a 3-year survivorship analysis. Spine 2000;25(2): 197–204.
[73] Van Tulder MW, Malmivaara A, Esmail R, et al. Exercise therapy for low back pain. Cochrane Database Syst Rev 2000;2:CD000335.
[74] Nagler W, Hausen HS. Conservative management of lumbar spinal stenosis: identifying patients likely to do well without surgery. Postgrad Med 1998;103(4):69–88.
[75] US Dept of Health and Human Services Agency for Healthcare Research and Quality. Treatment of degenerative lumbar spinal stenosis: summary. Evid Rep Technol Assess (Full Rep) 2001;32:1–5.
[76] Taylor CP, Gee NS, Kocsis JD, et al. A summary of mechanistic hypotheses of gabapentin pharmacology. Epilepsy Res 1998;29:233–49.
[77] Porter RW, Hibbert C. Calcitonin treatment for neurogenic claudication. Spine 1983;8(6): 585–92.
[78] Porter RW, Miller CG. Neurogenic claudication and root claudication treated with calcitonin: a double-blind trial. Spine 1988;13:1061–4.
[79] van Tulder MW, Scholten RJ, Koes BW, et al. Nonsteroidal anti-inflammatory drugs for low back pain: a systematic review within the framework of the Cochrane Collaboration Back Review Group. Spine 2000;25:2501–13.
[80] Psaty BM, Furber CD. COX-2 inhibitors—lessons in drug safety. N Engl J Med 2005;352: 1133–5.
[81] Cummins J, Lurie JD, Tosteson TD, et al. Descriptive epidemiology and prior health care utilization of patients in the spine patient outcomes research trials three observational cohorts. Spine 2006;31(7):806–14.

[82] Rydevik BL, Cohen DB, Kostuik JP. Spine epidural steroids for patients with spinal stenosis. Spine 1997;22:2313–7.

[83] Delport EG, Cucuzella AR, Marley JK, et al. Treatment of lumbar spinal stenosis with epidural steroid injections: a retrospective outcome study. Arch Phys Med Rehabil 2004; 85:479–84.

[84] Campbell MJ, Carron LY, Glassman SD, et al. Correlation of spinal canal dimensions to efficacy of epidural steroid injection in spinal stenosis. J Spinal Disord Tech 2007;20:168–71.

[85] Kapural L, Mekhail N, Bena J, et al. Value of the magnetic resonance imaging in patients with painful lumbar spinal stenosis undergoing lumbar epidural steroid injections. Clin J Pain 2007;23:571–5.

[86] Katz JN, Lipson ST, Larson MG, et al. The outcome of decompressive laminectomy for degenerative lumbar stenosis. J Bone Joint Surg Am 1991;73(6):809–16.

[87] Weinstein JN, Lurie JD, Torsteson TD, et al. Surgical versus nonsurgical treatment for lumbar degenerative spondylolisthesis. N Engl J Med 2007;356(22):2257–70.

[88] Herron L, Turner J, Clancy S, et al. The differential utility of the Minnesota multiphasic personality inventory: a predictor of outcome in lumbar laminectomy for disc herniation versus spinal stenosis. Spine 1986;11:847–50.

[89] Deen HG, Zimmerman RS, Lyons MK, et al. Analysis of early failures after lumbar decompressive laminectomy for spinal stenosis. Mayo Clin Proc 1995;70(1):33–6.

[90] Aalto TJ, Malmivaara A, Kovacs F, et al. Preoperative predictors for postoperative clinical outcome in lumbar spinal stenosis: systemic review. Spine 2006;31:E648–63.

[91] Martin BI, Mirza SK, Comstock BA, et al. Reoperation rates following lumbar spine surgery and the influence of spinal fusion procedures. Spine 2007;32:382–7.

[92] Weiner BK, Walker M, Brower RS, et al. Microdecompression for lumbar spinal canal stenosis. Spine 1999;24(21):2268–72.

[93] Lindsey DP, Swanson KE, Fuchs P, et al. The effects of an interspinous implant on the kinematics of the instrumented and adjacent levels in the lumbar spine. Spine 2003;28: 2192–7.

[94] Bono CM, Vaccaro AR. Interspinous process devices in the lumbar spine. J Spinal Disord Tech 2007;20:255–61.

[95] Zucherman JF, Hsu KY, Hartjen CA, et al. A multicenter, prospective, randomized trial evaluating the X STOP interspinous process decompression system for the treatment of neurogenic intermittent claudication: two-year follow-up results. Spine 2005;30(12):1351–8.

ELSEVIER
SAUNDERS

Clin Geriatr Med 24 (2008) 389–393

CLINICS IN
GERIATRIC
MEDICINE

Index

Note: Page numbers of article titles are in **boldface** type.